Guide to Me
1: Outline History, ~~~

a primer for Mental Health Workers

MARIANNE RICHARDS

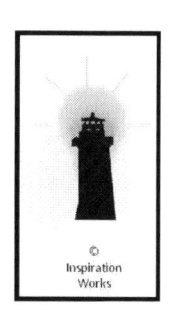

Inspiration Works

Copyright © 2017 Marianne Richards
All rights reserved.
ISBN: 151865519X
ISBN-13: 978-1518655197

MARIANNE RICHARDS

DEDICATION

Tim. Forever.

CONTENTS

	Page
Dedication	iii
Introduction	

1 Setting the Stage – Mad, Bad, Sane	5

HISTORY OF MENTAL ILLNESS

2 Mental Illness to 18th Century	11
3 Mental Illness to Late 19th Century	25
4 Mental Illness In 20th & 21st Century	33
5 Psychiatric Hospitals, Community Care	41

LEGISLATION & EDUCATION

6 Mental Health Act 1983	49
7 Proposed Mental Health Bill 2000	55
8 The World Health Organization	63

COMMUNITIES & SOCIAL EXCLUSION

9 Communities & Mental Illness	65
10 Stigma & Social Exclusion	71
11 Reducing Social Exclusion	85
12 Epilogue – Rachel's Challenge	89

Appx 1 Dr Parenti: Proposals for US Health Care	91

Further Reading	99
Glossary	101
About The Author	107
Index	109

MARIANNE RICHARDS

LIST OF ILLUSTRATIONS

Figure		page
1	Mental Illness- a Continuum	8
2	Mad, Bad or Criminally Insane	9
3	Patients at Bethlem Tormented by Visitors	13
4	Ancient Trepanned Skull	15
5	Medicine, Philosophy, Science and Nature	17
6	Medicinal Leech. C19th Glass Leech Case	19
7	Chained Patient in Bethlem Asylum	21
8	Hogarth's The Rake's Progress	23
9	Exterior of Bethlem Asylum, London	27
10	Morel's Degeneracy Theory	29
11	Electro-Convulsive Therapy & Medication	39
12	St John's Hospital, Chapel and Water Tower	43
13	Asylum Patient – Victorian drawing	45
14	St John's Hospital – Montage of Images	47
15	Proposed 2004 Bill - Flowchart	57
16	How a Bill Becomes Law	61
17	Perceptions of Individuals By Communities	67
18	Victoria Climbie Enquiry	69
19	David Bennett Enquiry	73
20	Contributory Factors to Mental Illness	79
21	Origin of Scapegoats	83
22	The Language of Stigma	86

OPINIONS EXPRESSED DO NOT NECESSARILY REFLECT THOSE OF REVIEWERS.

Text
Crown copyright material is reproduced with the permission of the Controller of HMSO and the Queen's Printer for Scotland. Websites for the information on the Mental Health Bill 2004 are stated at the end of the chapter on that subject.

Statistics reproduced on license from the National Statistics website: www.statistics.gov.uk

Summary of Mind proposals for the new Mental Health Bill written & approved by Mind media.

Images
Diagrams by Mole Graphics.

The following images [figure no + image reference] supplied by Wellcome Picture Library, under Creative Commons License http://wellcomeimages.org/. None of these images has been altered.
fig 3 M0017216; fig 4 M0005287; fig 6 L0014509 AND L0058201; fig 7 William Norris Chained in Bedlam L0006344; fig 8 William Hogarth, from The Rakes Progress V0016646; fig 9 Ext Bethlem Hospital L0011828; fig 11 ECT machine by Electron, L0065853 + L0070534; fig 13 L0026691.

Image of Victoria Climbie [RIP] Crown copyright, given under Creative Commons License from the following report: 'The Victoria Climbie Inquiry: Report of an Inquiry' Lord Laming. Jan 2003.'
https://www.gov.uk/government/uploads/system/uploads/attachment_data/file/273183/5730.pdf

Image of David Bennett [RIP] Crown copyright, given under Creative Commons License from the following report:
'Independent Inquiry into the death of David Bennett', Dec 2003
http://www.irr.org.uk/pdf/bennett_inquiry.pdf

St John's Asylum, photographs by author. Joint copyright author & the Buckinghamshire Collection.

'In the country of the blind, the one-eyed man is king'
Erasmus (1466-1536); also H G Wells 'The Country of the Blind'

1 SETTING THE STAGE – MAD, BAD, SANE
Content:
Terminology
Defining Sanity and insanity
Country of the Blind
Mad, Bad or Criminally Insane
Who Are the Mentally Ill

Terminology

When a class of people are marginalized, for whatever reason, one of the first things you will notice is negative language used to describe them. For example, in the 1930's the Nazis began to persecute Jews. I remember seeing extant footage of a small Jewish girl being asked her name and she replied, Jew Dog. This is the power of language not only to degrade but convince individuals of their worthlessness. Modern examples; a Manager who disliked me referred to me as cunning instead of using a nicer term like intelligent. Other staff members in remarking on my first published book - 'oh, your little booklet'; 'but you've only written one book"; 'you told me you were self published'.

Until the 19th century, the terms idiot, mad, lunatic and defective did not have pejorative overtones. They were used in times when little was known about the causes of mental illness. I have retained these terms for historic accuracy but do not wish readers to take offence. There is a deal of difference between deliberate insults and downgrading achievements.

Unfortunately, there are provocative words in common use about mentally ill persons, even in the press. The words maniac, lunatic [going out of use], crazy and nutter still have the power to dismay. Thanks to a long campaign by the Royal College of Psychiatrists, there are less displays of such language in the press, and less of the tendency to report suicides critically (including methodology). The use of mocking or derogatory words is a sure signpost of marginalization or what we now refer to as bullying (scapegoating).

Defining Sanity and Insanity

Now to explore the difference between those two extreme states, sanity and insanity. Unless we define what it means to be sane ('normal', neurotypical) we cannot diagnose deviations which indicate dysfunctional states.

These are some of the issues:

- do sanity and insanity exist
- how do we define mental illness
- is mental illness a social or community construct

Defining and recognizing mental illness is more difficult than you might imagine. Some professionals, even Psychiatrists, question whether sanity and insanity exist as states of mind or whether they are social constructs. You will understand more of this after reading the chapters on the history of mental illness. But once last thought before we leave this endlessly fascinating subject: the philosopher George Berkeley (1685-1753) posed an interesting question; 'if no one hears the sound of a tree falling in the forest, does that sound exist?' I am going to pose a question; does insanity exist, if there is no one to observe it?

Imagine an eccentric man alone on an island; could his extraordinary perceptions be said to be sane? If someone with different perceptions joins him, who is sane and who deluded - or are their realities both valid? In which case, how many people need to live on this island, before sanity or insanity (meaning, 'out of touch with reality') can be defined? Following is a another way of expressing this, in the metaphor 'the country of the blind'.

Country of the Blind

This tale is retold in the H. G. Wells short story, The Country of the Blind. A man lost in the mountains finds himself in a strange community where everyone is blind. Being sighted, he believes himself superior and wants to be King. As he begins to describe the 'wonders' he sees, people disbelieve him and become angry. They accuse him of lying. Instead of becoming King, he is forced to run away. But hunger forces him to seek out the tribe. He pretends he can't see and is accepted. He falls in love with a girl but when he again starts to speak of what he sees, she is afraid. The community believe he is mad. Their wise men suggest the only cure is to rid him of the cause of his misery – the organs he calls eyes. I won't spoil the ending in case you want to read it, but this is an excellent metaphor.

No one can be certain what someone else is thinking because no one has the ability to enter someone else's mind. Human communication is a crude tool and it is no wonder that the world's conflicts begin with misunderstandings.

We could define 'going mad' as having extraordinary perceptions which other people do not share. But, if this is true, the religious ecstasies reported by hermits or anchorites might be considered madness and not divine inspiration. People in solitary confinement report hallucinations and on rejoining society are often reported to have undergone marked changes in perception. But if you suggested to someone steeped in religious or mystical practice that their vision was only a hallucination and should be treated with

Haloperidol, you would most certainly offend them.

So our problem of sanity is one of perception. This is a profound question indeed. You are not merely diagnosing a patient but asking an existential question - whose reality is real, whose perception or spiritual nuances are valid and who decides?

Mad, Bad or Criminally Insane

Not so long ago we had a spate of moral panics about murder; which confused criminal acts with acts committed by people with serious mental conditions such as paranoid schizophrenia or personality disorder. There are relatively few murders committed by mentally ill people, most being committed by sane criminals. Such judgements cannot be made by laymen. Although their behaviour defies moral codes, none of the following were ruled by the Courts of Justice to be criminally insane:

- Eric Harris and Dylan Klebold - assassinated 13 innocent young students at Columbine High School, America
- Harold Shipman – GP who poisoned an unknown number of his patients. Over 887 deaths were investigated in the public enquiry of which he is suspected of killing at least 260.
- Armin Meiwes – a cannibal who advertised for a willing victim on the internet and found one in Bernd Jurgen Brandes. Meiwes was imprisoned for murder, but not considered insane.
- Ian Brady – child killer of the 1950's, who with his partner Myra Hindley (now deceased) murdered several children and buried them on the Yorkshire moors. Brady was born psychopathic, that is he was born without the part of mind we call conscience or morality. Brady was sent to Broadmoor where he still lives, now in his 80's.

Those considered criminally insane [i.e. diminished responsibility due to a diagnosed mental illness] receive what few treatments are available. Forensic mentally ill patients are usually sentenced to hospitals for the criminally insane, such as Broadmoor or Carstairs, rather than prisons.

Current thinking recognizes there is a great deal of difference between breaking the law whilst sane and committing crimes during an episode of mental illness. The difference is one of intent. Whilst the above deliberately set out to murder, they were ruled by the Courts to be sane when they made their, albeit horrific, decisions.

Who Are the Mentally Ill

All of us suffer stress and nearly 25% of the population will be diagnosed with a mental illness at some point in our lives. I find it amusing that I was one of few mental health workers who could prove my sanity; having had a breakdown and been discharged from a mental hospital.

Illness of the mind is a common experience, not something that afflicts an imagined sub-species of human. Mental illness is extremely common. the only reason this is not common knowledge is that it remains a taboo subject across the world. In the NHS, it is frowned upon for mental health professionals to admit to being afflicted with mental illness, as if somehow denigrates their position. This attitude is understandable in trainees. All trainees are at first nervous of their subject, afraid of making errors, until time and experience allows them to relax their view. But this attitude of 'them' and 'us' is sheer hypocrisy, does not help to reduce stigma and in fact degrades mentally ill patients.

1:4 people will be diagnosed with depressive illness and 1:25 with schizophrenia. Many more attend GP's for physical symptoms connected with mental distress: skin problems, backache, physical aches and tiredness, emotional disorders. So why is it that people seemingly happy to talk to a GP about intimate body parts but reluctant to talk about emotional problems, disturbances to perception (hallucinations) or other signs of mental aberration. You might discuss such symptoms with a loved one, but talking outside family, at least in the UK, is also taboo. In the US people do not have such hesitation. Revealing a visit to a psychiatrist is more likely to trigger a request for his/her contact details than negative reaction.

There are many reasons for stigma; fear, lack of knowledge, bad press, fear of prognosis, shame. There are many false perceptions about mental illness being lifelong, whereas many symptoms are controlled by medication, some have but one episode, others irregular episodes or, in the case of depression, there may be a single episode and no more.

Even with the plethora of information of information available in this electronic age, a huge proportion of the public only become aware of the fact of mental illness through sensational headlines. Thankfully this is changing due to liaison between the media and the Royal College of Psychiatrists. Far more murders are committed by so-called sane people (bad) than by mentally ill persons ('mad').

Some individuals become dangerous through their mental disorders; personality disorder, some forms of schizophrenia, paraphilia or paedophilia. None of these states are yet curable. The only way of ensuring very ill (psychotic) patients receive treatment is compulsory hospitalization. Many professionals do not class stress as mental illness though it is an illness of the mind. It is useful to consider a continuum. This is not an 'always and forever' line; everyone fluctuates along that line according to, environment, genetic factors, stress.

Figure 1   Mental Illness – a Continuum

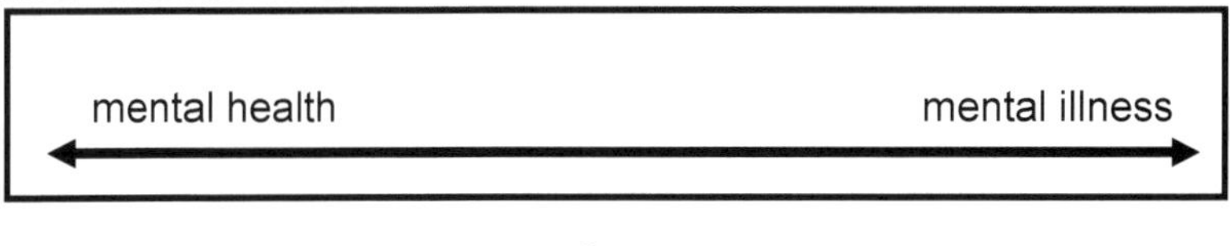

mental health ←——————————————→ mental illness

Figure 2 Mad, Bad or Criminally Insane

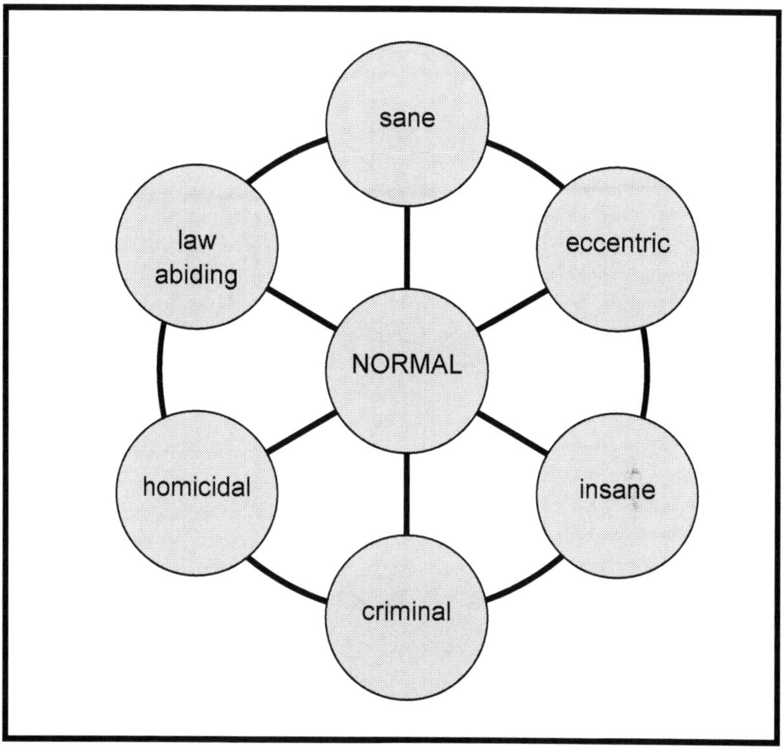
sane
eccentric
insane
criminal
homicidal
law
abiding
NORMAL

Key Learning

- Terminology – derogatory language is used to marginalise
- Sanity and insanity – there is no hard borderline
- Mad, bad or criminally insane – depend on legal code of society
- Commonality of mental illness – anyone can develop mental illness

'The past is a foreign country; we do things differently there.'
L P Hartley, the Go Between
****

<u>A Short History of Medicine</u> [from The Quote Garden]
2000 B.C. - "Here, eat this root."
1000 B.C. - "That root is heathen, say this prayer."
1850 A.D. - "That prayer is superstition, drink this potion."
1940 A.D. - "That potion is snake oil, swallow this pill."
1985 A.D. - "That pill is ineffective, take this antibiotic."
2000 A.D. - "That antibiotic is artificial. Here, eat this root."
http://www.quotegarden.com/medical.html

2 MENTAL ILLNESS TO 18TH CENTURY

Content:
Context of Mental Illness
Primitive Belief
Ancient Trepanning
Ancient Greeks and Divine Retribution
Hippocrates and Medical Reasoning
Other Ancient Treatments for Mental Illness
Medieval Belief
The Sixteenth Century
New For Old – Lazar Houses Revamped as Asylums
Ship of Fools
Treatment in Early Asylums

In the 1920's sex and contraception were taboo subjects. The Victorian considered sex as functional, purely for procreation and a duty for women within a marriage context. Marie Stopes' pioneering sex therapy book, Married Love, overturned that view. Dr Stopes advocated sexual and contraceptive advice and was greatly reviled in her time. It is only with hindsight her pioneer work has been recognized. Stopes clinics are now worldwide, offering happier marriages, better attitudes to women and less poverty through overlarge families.

Context of Mental Illness
When considering a history of any field, it is vital to gain a rounded view by attempting to understand the attitude of those who lived at the time. The field of mental illness is no different. Sadly, there are still people who equate mental illness with moral or social degeneracy, which is a Victorian view. Balancing this are those who view mental illness as a gift, for example in the

context of more sensitivity to spirituality, creativity or ability to empathize with others.

Some early treatments are still considered effective, for example the light and sleep temples of the ancient world and Asylums sited in peaceful gardens with plenty of fresh air. The old Roman treatment of electric eels is practiced in the modern form of ECT, though this is rarely used. Even if treatments are now considered defunct or even dangerous, it is vital to have a knowledge of where modern treatments originated and the thinking behind them. All good practitioners will have an interest in the history of their subject. In the West we re-hash ancient therapies but rarely acknowledge this fact. Many treatment regimes might appear bizarre, horrific and outlandish to us, but in their day they were considered cutting edge. Our own descendants will no doubt consider modern treatments inhumane, strange and primitive.

Mal Practice

And here is another controversy which needs airing. Sometimes patient vulnerability has 'given license for cruelty or torture in the name of treatment. I am sure then, as now, not all treatment given the patient was for their good but for the pleasure of others. Look at the next image which shows Bethlem Hospital visitors making mock of patients. We are imperfect creatures. Because someone bears the title therapist it does not make them saintly (consider Harold Shipman or nurses who kill patients). I remember in the 1990's seeing patients made to wash senior staff cars and nurses mocking bizarre behaviour. It is to be hoped you will be on your guard for such malpractice throughout your career. Denial is a sure way of prolonging such behaviour, as is failing to report malpractice of seniors.

Primitive Belief

It is impossible to know early man's inner thinking processes and archaeologists can only make educated guesses through examining findings at grave sites, early written or oral traditions.

We assume that, in early times, strange behaviour was not seen as the result of an illness but punishments sent by an angry or jealous god. The appropriate person to deal with this was a priest or shaman, who was an intermediary between the gods and members of the tribe or community . This powerful person would either rule the tribe or be very close to the ruler.. He would make rituals and sacrifices to appease the deity, hoping to ward off suffering to the rest of the community. Of course, if this priest failed, he faced death or casting out, for like modern Doctors, he was responsible for ensuring the health and well being of the tribe.

figure 3 Patients at Bethlem Hospital Tormented by Visitors

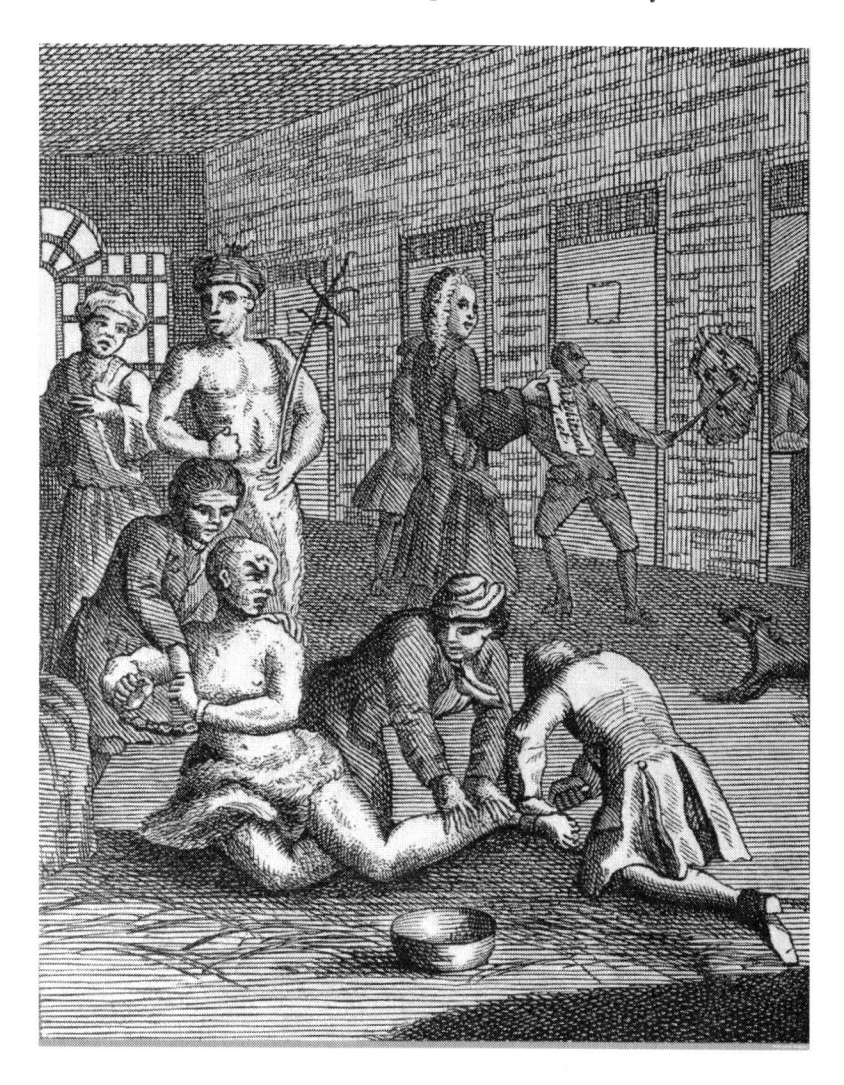

The afflicted person or scapegoat might shoulder blame for all that went wrong in the community; loss of crops or unexplained deaths. These losses were not attributed to natural disaster or disease but to angry gods inflicting punishment. Human or animal sacrifices were made to appease these gods by the giving of blood (symbolic life).

Primitive people drew pictures on cave walls as acts of faith; creating the conditions for successful hunts with these symbolic representations. The linking of real to imagined events was an intellectual leap. Of course there could be other interpretations for primitive art. When man began to adopt farming and began to live in large communities there would be more free time to spend on making art. Perhaps we can consider decorative art as an early form of home improvement and celebratory art the equivalent of gaining a certificate or football trophy. The study of primitive culture is called anthropology, a fascinating and alluring subject.

However, there are many interpretations for historic events.

Ancient Trepanning

Many trepanned Neolithic human skulls have been found; the earliest examples of crude psycho-surgery. Trepanning was the process of cutting a circular hole in the skull to allow evil spirits to leave. Or could it be that powerful deities might be induced to enter a man, endowing him with powerful magic.

Archaeologists noticed bone growth around such holes in primitive skulls which indicate that, astonishingly, many survived this operation. This practice was widespread from the Stone Age to 5th century BC and through many cultures including Ancient Greeks and the American Indians.

Ancient Greeks and Divine Retribution

The Greeks were sophisticated thinkers who were among the first to look more deeply into the question of judgement and the reasons behind natural disasters. Rather than a greedy wish for meat and blood, they attributed gods with moral justice. Their gods sent dilemmas for the afflicted person to solve and allowed the god might be satisfied with atonement instead of death. However, Greek tragedy always contains death or someone being sent mad. It is the ancient equivalent of The Terminator. It reflects a Greek love of drama. These tragedies were performed on huge outdoor public stages. The voice of conscience was acted by a group of actors called the Chorus. The players wore symbolic masks to depict their character. When you read this tale, remember these ancient Greek truths:
- disobeying a god is a sin punishable by the Furies
- matricide (killing a mother) is a sin punishable by death
- (consider the Furies a kind of paparazzi)

figure 4 Ancient Trepanned Skull

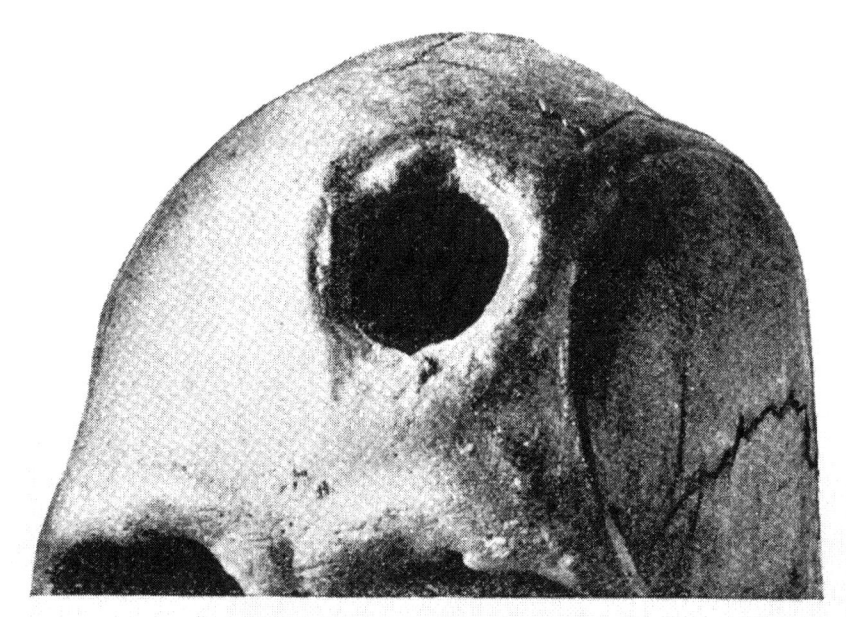

Abb. 49. Trepanierter Schädel von Neu-Britannien
(K. k. Naturhistorisches Hofmuseum in Wien [nach Zdekauer])

Myth of the House of Agamemnon
The god Apollo orders Orestes, son of King Agamemnon & Queen Clytemnestra, to put his mother to death. This sentence was set because the Queen and her lover Aegisthus had murdered King Agamemnon. Orestes agonizes. If he kills Clytemnestra he will disobey the goddess Athena's law; all matricide is punishable by death. If he refuses, he will be hounded by the Furies. Orestes, helped by his sister Elektra, kills Clytemnestra and Aegisthus. Orestes is then inflicted with madness by the Furies. As he is nearing death, Athena intervenes and the curse of the House of Agamemnon is lifted.

So, centuries before Sigmund Freud, the Greeks had discovered how mental conflict (moral dilemmas) results in temporary loss of reason (stress or temporary insanity). Once conflicts had been worked through (using psycho or mind therapy) the sufferer would recover. This is not far from modern drama therapy, in which patients 'act' out problems and re-enact events with positive endings.

Hippocrates and Medical Reasoning

Greek philosopher Hippocrates is considered the father of modern medicine. He made a study of illnesses of the mind two thousand years ago. Far ahead of his time, he concluded madness was 'no more divine nor sacred than other diseases but has a natural cause'. This was a landmark. Hippocrates was first to overturn the conventional view of madness as punishment by gods. Pre-empting modern medical science, Hippocrates examined his patients and distinguished three types of mental disorder:

- brain fever
- mania
- melancholia

These terms remained in use to the nineteenth century. Indeed, the term mania is still in use today. The term melancholy was widely used in the 16th century. William Shakespeare's play Hamlet contains what is considered an accurate description of melancholia – what we now call depressive illness. In Victorian times melancholia became fashionable, the penchant of poets who dosed themselves with laudanum, opium or cocaine for spiritual relief and to enhance their creative powers. To a certain extent this remains 'sexy' in certain circles, as have smoking, drug rehab and drinking.

Hippocrates, Galen and their followers believed the human body was made of four elements called humours or vital fluids. If these fluids were out of balance, he or she became ill. To date neither psychological nor chemical analysis proved the existence of humours, though belief persists.

Figure 5 Medicine, Philosophy, Science & Nature

Mandela

Throughout the ages, circular symmetries (mandelas) were believed to have magical and healing properties. This diagram illustrates mandelas from nature, alchemy and early medicine.

Illness was believed caused by imbalances in the vital fluids (humours). Doctors treated patients by 're-balancing' these fluids - using leeches (blood letting), induced fever or cold. Thus, symmetry was restored and the patient recovered.

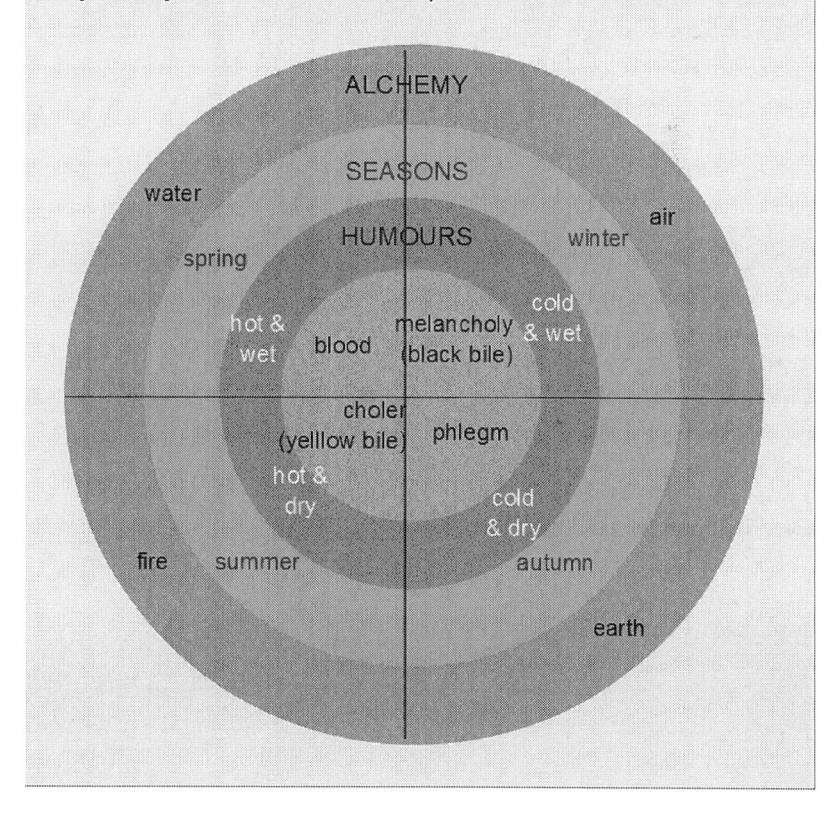

ALCHEMY
SEASONS
HUMOURS

water
air
spring
winter
hot & wet
blood
melancholy (black bile)
cold & wet
choler (yelllow bile)
phlegm
hot & dry
cold & dry
fire
summer
autumn
earth

I have depicted the crossover of medicine, science, philosophy and nature (see Mandela diagram). From the outer circle are:
1. the elemental symbols in alchemy [air, earth, fire, water]
2. the four seasons – each fixed with certain religious rites
3. four physical states, caused by imbalance of the vital fluids
4. four humours / vital fluids (blood, phlegm, black bile, yellow bile

A mandela is a magic symbol used in holistic medicine to represent the perfect harmony between mind, body and spirit. To restore patients to health, it is the Physician's work to balance the elements. Early treatments for doing this might seem bizarre, but were practiced into the 18th century. The mainstays of early medicine were

☹ purging – through inducing vomiting
☹ bloodletting - using lancets or leeches

Leeches secrete a solution which prevents blood from clotting. Leeches can be sent into difficult to reach areas of the body. You might find it surprising that leeches have been re-introduced into modern surgery, to prevent blockage to blood flow, vital in cosmetic operations. 21st century sensibilities require leeches to be encased in plastic shields which hide their hideous appearance. Leech dress, as it were, is by no means new. See the drawing of a medicinal leech with a nineteenth century glass leech case.

Other Ancient Treatments for Mental Illness

The Greek philosopher Plato said madmen (historic term) ought to be locked away at home. Such practice was widespread until the early nineteenth century England before the rise of public Asylums enabled relatives to dump unwanted progeny and forget them.

Romans were familiar with and tolerant of depressive illness. They treated this condition with warm baths, music and well lighted rooms. Such treatments would still be recognized as beneficial. Ancient Greeks and Romans had access to sleep temples where soporific herbs were given as curative aids to rest and sleep. In modern times, a sleep treatment called modified narcosis was used for patients with severe depressive illness, in danger of exhaustion through lack of sleep. Narcosis was induced by drugs.

Romans reportedly used electric eels to shock patients out of madness a treatment used in Bethlem Hospital to the 19th century, with patients lowered into a tub of eels. This ancient treatment may be a precursor of 20th century electric shock treatment (ECT) where an electric current is introduced through electrodes attached either side of the brain. ECT is still used although under strict guidelines. No one knows how this works but it does, in schizophrenia or depression not responding to other treatment.

Figure 6   Drawing of a Medicinal Leech &

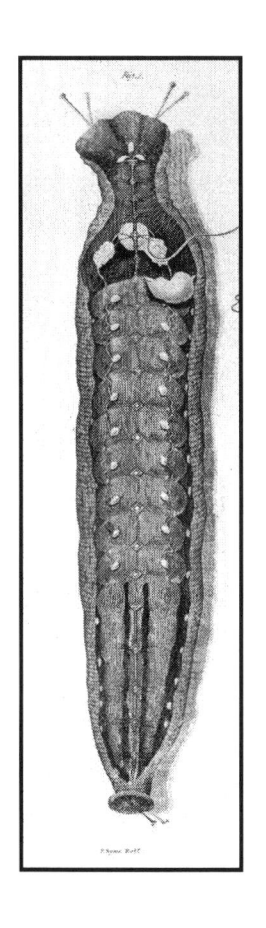

19th century Glass Leech Case

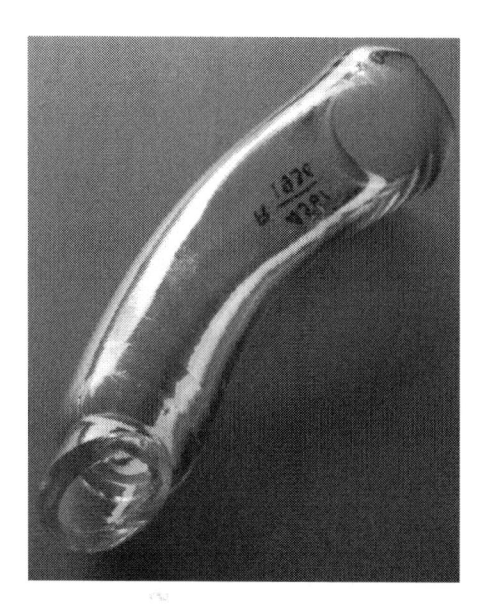

Medieval Belief

By medieval times, there was a mix of beliefs between divine retribution witchcraft and more enlightened attitudes toward idiots and lunatics [historic terms]. Idiots were deemed to be born defective, lunatics to have been afflicted with disorder during their lifetime. The word lunacy reflects an early belief that the moon affected sanity.

Belief in witchcraft lasted until late into the 17th century. Sick people and animals were considered possessed by evil spirits as a result of curses placed by witches (human servants of the devil). The Church, concerned at immoral sexual activity between monks and nuns were reluctant to put blame on their ordained servants, which would look bad for the church, and therefore claimed it was the Devil who incited the nuns and monks to passion. The book The Devils of Loudon by Aldous Huxley (and movie of the same name by Ken Russell) is a graphic depiction of this time in history.

In contrast to this, read the interesting article by David and Christine Roffe in the British Medical Journal about Emma de Beston [see further reading]. Emma de Beston's case is one of few surviving accounts of a medieval woman brought before a local Inquisition for lunacy. Inquisitions were special courts, under the jurisdiction of the Pope, set up to try witches and had immense power. But Emma Beston's is a rare case of someone being treated fairly by an Inquisition. The court prevented her wicked relatives from depriving her of liberty and her property. Although Beston never recovered her reason, the court enabled her to regain her property and access to services for her welfare. This case is a model for fairness which Roffe interestingly compares with less favourable patient experiences of the Care in the Community Act of the 1990's, a view with which I would agree, having worked in the mental health field at this time. It was not all enlightenment and fairness however.

Bethlehem Hospital (known as Bethlem or Bedlam) was an infamous insane Asylum set up through public subscription in 1377. This establishment set out to lock up the insane out of harm's way (and out of sight of their families). An early Asylum might incarcerate those with (using historic terms):

- shaking palsy (epilepsy, cerebral palsy)
- mental defectives (genetic causes or head injuries)
- wanderers (tramps, , prostitutes)
- master-less men (itinerants)

The Sixteenth Century

By the 16th Century, mental illness was commonly considered an illness or malady. Roy Porter describes the changing view of society towards a 'more philosophical view' and quotes Descartes; 'reason can rescue man from insanity'. Madness was nevertheless still regarded as a curse.

Figure 7 Chained Patient, Bethlem Asylum

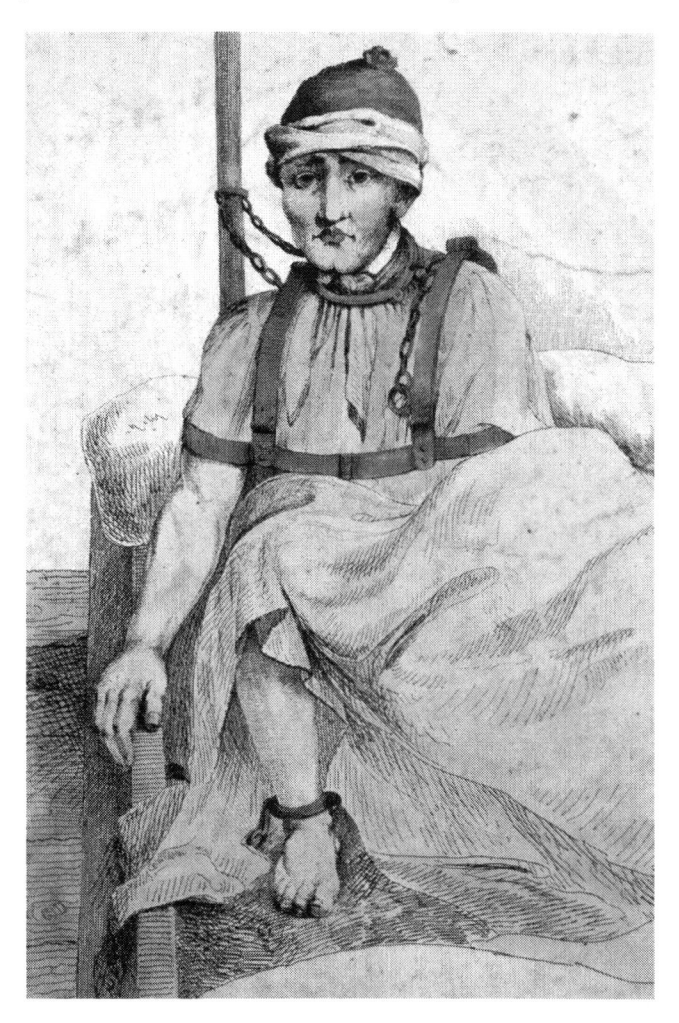

The cure was prayer and bible reading. This perception conveniently helped the church maintain a hold over frightened communities. However, monasteries and nunneries began to provide shelter for the insane in their communities, where inmates were tolerated.

New For Old – Lazar Houses Revamped as Asylums

In his excellent if a little obscure book Madness and Civilization (written in the 1960's) Michel Foucault makes interesting parallels between religious fervour and the exclusion of anyone perceived as sinners. Leprosy had been a scourge from the Middle Ages. Thousands of Lazar Houses had been set up where lepers could find refuge after being forcibly excluded from their communities. Cruel popular belief dictated that leprosy was a punishment for sins and to cast out a leper was an act of piety. As Foucault ironically remarks, 'the sinner who abandons the leper .. opens his [the sinner's] way to heaven'.

By the 16th Century this policy of social exclusion had by accident curtailed the spread of leprosy, which is spread by contact. By the end of the century, Lazar Houses were virtually empty. What better place to exclude a whole new raft of society than these crumbling buildings across Europe. Those considered outcasts found themselves socially and spiritually excluded 'for their own good'. Foucault sees the ironic link between the their exclusion and eventual spiritual re-generation through being placed outside stressful society.

Ship of Fools

'Ship of fools' (historic term) was a curious treatment, popular during the Renaissance. Alongside the forcible stuffing of the insane into ex-Lazar Houses, the good citizens found another convenient way of tidying up their streets. There was a supposed affinity between calmness and the sea. Foucault describes how madmen would be given into the care of mariners who would take their cargo of insane on long voyages. These were ordinary trading ships and ordinary seamen, not Physicians.

In effect some lunatics (historic terms) did recover, probably through the fresh air, removal from humiliations of daily life, regular food and relative calm. In mental illness excess stimuli [noise, confusion, lack of routine] are counter-productive to creating the calm required for confused minds to recover. The other side of the coin were lonely deaths, far from family and country. One wonders how many were 'lost at sea' (put over the side) if mariners could not cope with bizarre behaviour. Casting overboard ill human cargo was common during the slave trade. Ship of Fools became an allegorical term with romantic as well macabre aspects, written into folklore. Read Foucault's splendid book for more detail.

figure 8 Wm Hogarth, Rake's Progress – Tom Rakewell in Bedlam

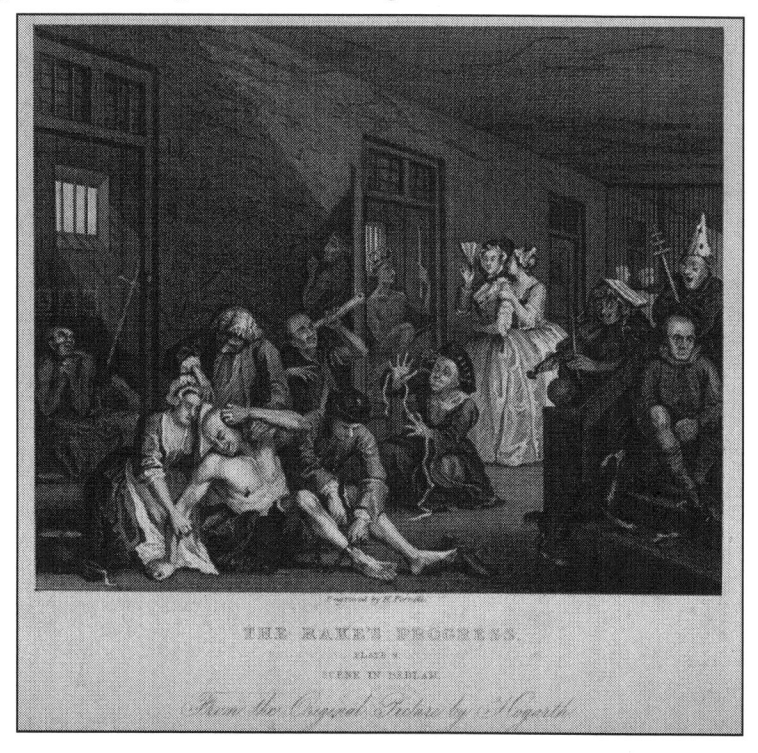

Treatment in Early Asylums

Although mental illness was still not regarded as treatable in the same way as physical illness, it was recognized that something had to be done. When Bethlem was built, no inmate was expected to recover and most patients died within its walls deserted by friends, family and community. Male and female patients were kept in appalling conditions, naked, restrained or chained and sleeping on straw. Vomiting and purging were administered to reduce strength and keep patients controlled. Asylum Doctors formulated patent quack medicines which patients were forced to buy. Some patients were discharged and given a badge as a license to beg in the surrounding villages. In a cruel reversal, they were expected to repay the cost of their treatment in Bethlem from their earnings.

On Sundays the public paid 1d to view patients as an entertainment yet visitors interested in patient welfare were discouraged. 17th century artist William Hogarth's series of drawings The Rake's Progress graphically depict Bethlem (see next page), with Tom Rakewell finally succumbing to madness and death. The following barbaric treatments were administered to patients. I indicate in brackets how the treatments were believed to have worked;

- put patient in tub with electric eels [shocks into wellness]
- draw blood [excess blood on the brain causes madness]
- lower patient in water inside box drilled with holes [fear of death forced patient to sanity]
- spinning the patient on a stool [shaking the brain into sanity]
- cutting off clitoris [sexual organs caused melancholia]

An 1820 Act of Parliament at last made it compulsory to have medically qualified practitioners in attendance at Asylums. Previously Asylums had been run by Superintendents who were not qualified but experienced in dealing with inmate behaviour.

****

Key Learning

- historic context of mental illness & treatments - extant attitudes reveal thinking behind perceived treatment and 'cure'..
- historic remedies often rehashed - ancient therapies are often re-invented but this is rarely acknowledged.
- interpretation of history - speculation based on world archaeology
- popularised traits – tendency for aspects of mental illness to become an accessory; melancholia, in 'rehab', blasé about drug taking.

'The sole purpose of human existence is to kindle a light in the darkness of mere being.'
Carl Jung, Memories, Dreams & Reflections

3 MENTAL ILLNESS TO LATE 19TH CENTURY

Content:
Psychiatry in the 18th Century
The York Retreat 1796
Degeneration (Benedict Morel 1809 – 1873)
Growing Power of Psychiatrists
Meaning of Asylum
Poets and Melancholia
The Rise of Psychosurgery
Early Psychological Approaches – Talking Cures
Charcot [1835 - 1893] & Breuer [1842 - 1925]
Sigmund Freud [1856 1939]
Carl Jung [1875 - 1961] - Analytical Psychology
Carl Jung - Analytical Psychology
Behaviourists; Pavlov, Watson, Thorndike & Skinner

Psychiatry in the 18th Century

By the early 18th century madness was commonly viewed as a disease of the mind. In 1788 King George III was diagnosed with mental illness and received psychological therapy at home. He is now believed to have suffered arsenic poisoning.

Doctors began to explore psychological links between the nervous system, senses and intellect. Studies were made of shaking palsy (epilepsy), tics, hallucinations and aphasia (disturbance of the senses).

Phrenology, study of personality by examining head bumps was briefly popular before being discredited. The inventors were anatomists.

The York Retreat 1796

Quaker William Tuke set up an institution based on moral therapy where patients lived-in with the staff. Tuke witnessed a fellow Quaker dying in an Asylum and was determined no one should suffer in that way again. His patients were rewarded for good behaviour and punished for bad to restoring the mind through moral and bible therapy. Tuke's Retreat in York is still active [The Retreat] though not in its original form. It was a forerunner of modern sanctuaries such as Maytree in London. Suicidal people can stay four days, an opportunity for quiet retreat with access to therapists.

Degeneration (Benedict Morel 1809 – 1873)

Morel's believed that certain families showed signs which designated they were on a downward spiral to madness. He outlined the stages as:

- alcohol and opiate addiction
- prostitution and sexual degeneracy
- criminality
- insanity
- imbecility
- sterility

Decades before genes and genetic inheritance were discovered, Morel believed birth defects to be the cause of imbecility (historic term). Morel may have been way out by today's standards but consider his degeneracy theory in the light of genetics. In looking at the history of mental illness we must turn back again and again to context. This was decades before genes were discovered, so Morel was very much a pioneer.

Morel believed degeneracy was due to drug or alcohol abuse, diseases like malaria or moral sickness. He believed the diseased family would eventually become sterile and die out naturally and mercifully. His beliefs bore more of a resemblance to natural selection than the evil advocates of eugenics who preached racial purity through mass slaughter of ' inferior' beings (i.e. anyone outside their group).

Growing Power of Psychiatrists

This is a key time for Psychiatry. Superintendents were not qualified in medicine but exposure to the inmates of Asylums gave them practical experience in managing patient behaviour. In pre-medication times patients could be violent and unruly.

The Government began to introduce laws for the treatment of the mentally ill. By 1845 every county had to build an Asylum and by 1890 two medical certificates to be signed before anyone could be detained. These measures were brought in to stem cruel practices like dumping morel defectives (historic term for pregnant single women and itinerants) in Asylums when these people had no symptoms of mental illness. This practice had given carte blanche to unscrupulous people seeking early inheritance by ridding themselves of relatives. These patients gradually became institutionalized and forgotten. The Victorians favoured large institutions. Asylums held up to 1000 patients in mini towns. The acres of land surrounding Asylums contained kitchens, chapels, laundries, industrial units and gardens. Patients were expected to take a trade. Many creatives ended their lives in Bethlem, including Richard Dadd and William Cowper.

figure 9 Exterior Bethlem Asylum, London.

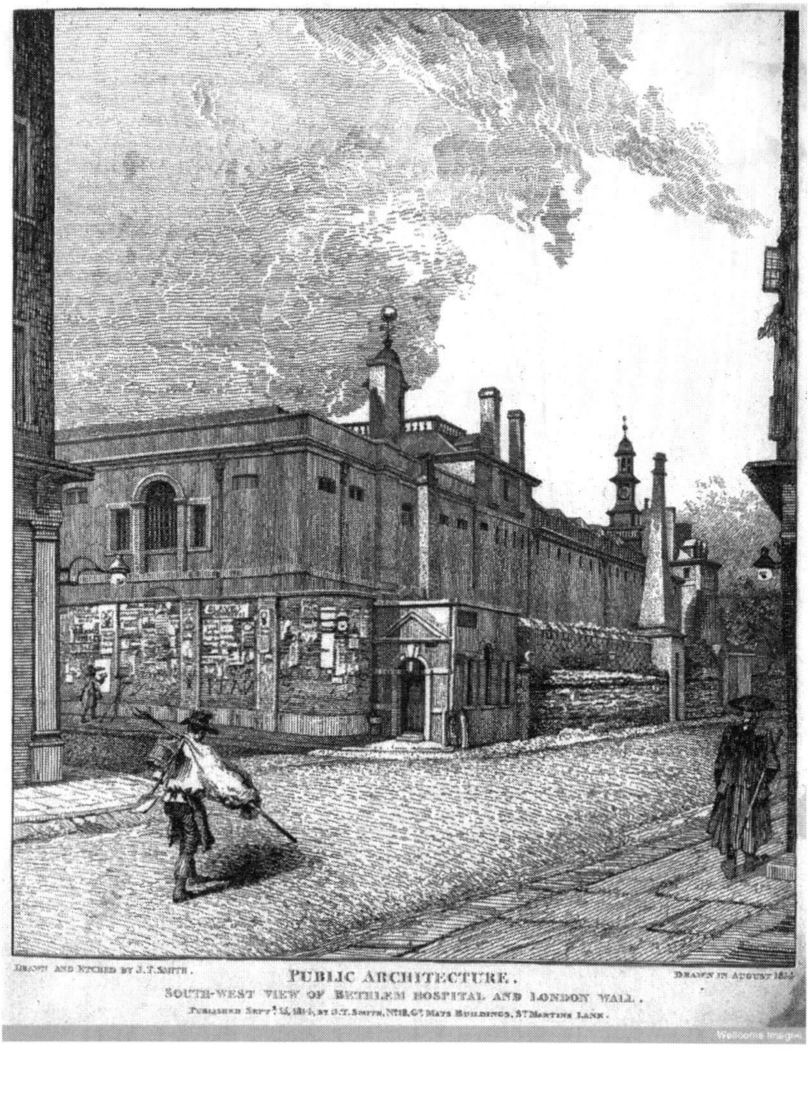

Rich patients were treated either in private madhouses (run by Doctors) or at home. Reformer Robert Gardiner Hill ran the Lincoln Asylum where restraints and strait jackets were replaced with activity-centred therapy, a wholesome diet and exercise. Unsurprisingly this regime proved successful. Art therapies were available to patients and these remain popular.

Meaning of Asylum

Asylum meant place of refuge. My photographs of St John's Hospital, Stone are in the archives of the Centre for Buckinghamshire Studies in Aylesbury but I have included a montage of images for interest.

Poets and Melancholia

By Late Victorian times, melancholy [depression] had become fashionable in artistic circles and among the public who adored them. There is an enduring romantic image of pale and languid artistic types sitting among idyllic sylvan scenes whilst partaking of laudanum [a form of opium] to enhance their writings - Keats, Shelley, Byron, Dickens, Coleridge; even abolitionist William Wilberforce. The mildly 'mad' image was particularly attached to Lord Byron famously referred to by a lover as 'mad, bad and dangerous to know'. The truth was less delightful as there were frequent deaths from arsenic or laudanum, taken to get the popular tuberculosis look of pallid flesh and large eyes.

The Rise of Psychosurgery

Phineas Gage – Discovery of the Frontal Lobes

In 1848 an event took place which was to radically alter treatment of behavioural disorders. Phineas Gage, a railroad worker, was exploding rocks with dynamite when a charge went off unexpectedly and drove a 25mm steel rod into his brain. Immediately after this horrific accident Gage became unconscious and had epileptic fits. Although he survived 11 years after the accident he became aggressive to an extent that his friends said they no longer recognized him. Gage was studied by many eminent doctors of the day. After his death, his brain was examined and scientists pinpointed the damaged frontal lobe area as the cause of the permanent change to his personality. These findings lead to an infamous operation called lobotomy or leucotomy, where the frontal lobes of the brain were severed with a sharp implement. Gage's skull is now in the Warren Anatomical Museum of Harvard Medical School.

Early Psychological Approaches – Talking Cures

Modern therapists began to revert to Hippocrates view, that mental illness stems from inner problems rather than being the result of external forces or environment.

Figure 10 Morel's Degeneracy Theory

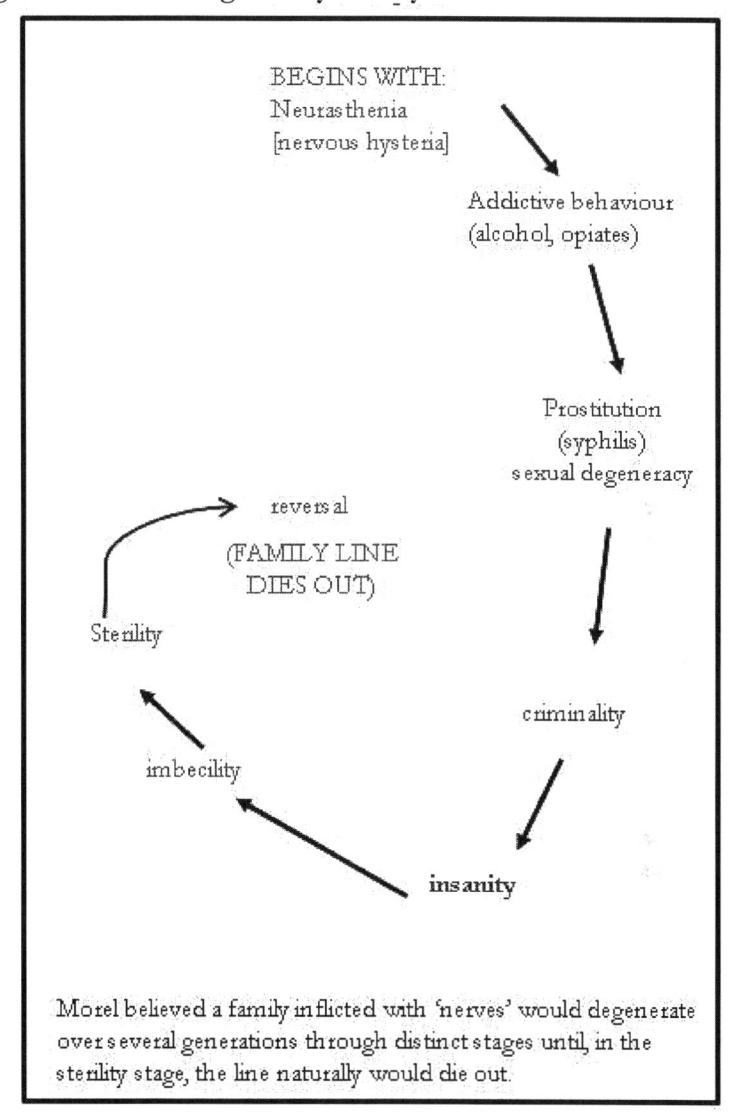

BEGINS WITH:
Neurasthenia
[nervous hysteria]

↓

Addictive behaviour
(alcohol, opiates)

↓

Prostitution
(syphilis)
sexual degeneracy

↓

criminality

↓

insanity

→ imbecility

→ Sterility

reversal
(FAMILY LINE DIES OUT)

Morel believed a family inflicted with 'nerves' would degenerate over several generations through distinct stages until, in the sterility stage, the line naturally would die out.

Freud introduced a way of approaching this by using analysis or structured talking rather than medication. Talking cure was a term coined by one of Sigmund Freud's patients Anna O, describing how Freud cured her of her neurosis. This term became generic for all the psychological therapies.

Charcot [1835 - 1893] & Breuer [1842 - 1925]

Jean Martin Charcot worked with patients diagnosed with hysterical paralyses referred to as conversion disorders and now very rare. Charcot discovered hypnotic suggestion successfully freed patients from physical symptoms. His colleague Joseph Breuer allowed patients to talk under hypnosis and discovered this freed them from neuroses. Freud collaborated with both men early in his career. Breuer and Freud named the hypnotic effect catharsis or cathexis (Greek for cleansing or discharging).

Sigmund Freud [1856 1939]

Sigmund Freud and his follower Carl Jung were the founding fathers of psychological therapies. Freud furthered his work with Charcot and Breuer by discovering symbolic meanings which revealed themselves during the cathexis (freeing) of hypnosis. Freud later abandoned hypnosis in favour of the view that the therapeutic relationship (relationship between therapist and patient) gave the cure, not the cathexis. Freud developed the method called psychoanalysis (psyche being Greek for mind) in which symbolic meanings were analysed. His life work was to understand the subconscious.

Carl Jung [1875 - 1961] - Analytical Psychology

Although Carl Jung was an early follower of Freud he eventually split and founded his own theory of analytical psychology. Jung's life work was based on understanding the personality. Jung coined the terms introvert and extrovert to describe two major aspects of personality

- introvert - inner reflective
- extrovert - worldly and sociable

Jung was deeply interested in philosophy and studied world mythology, spiritual and religious beliefs. He came to the conclusion there were unconscious links between people because similar stories occurred across cultures and through the ages worldwide.

Common character types in the myths were hero, wise man and fool, each of whom has a specific journey. In the hero myth a man is born of a virgin and is first sacrificed, then resurrected to save his people. The hero myth has commonality in many religions. If you want to read more I recommend:

- The Larousse Book of World Mythology

- Standard Stories from the Opera
- Man and his Symbols (Jung's book)

Jung believed that we all have archetypical characters (archetypes) within our personality. Through studying patients he came to believe that neurosis was a failure of the patient to integrate their archetypes. Naturally, the work of a Jungian Analyst was to help the patient discover and integrate all aspects of their personality, a process Jung referred to as individuation. Through individuation a patient becomes a mature person.

Jung's study of archetypes lead to consideration of the carrier which allowed memories to be retained across generations. He called this carrier the collective unconscious, that part of mind which retains ancient tribal memories, traditions and myths. The term unconscious refers to the fact that we are not only aware of archetypal memories except in certain conditions:

- symbolism of dreams
- de ja vue – instinctive feelings we have been somewhere before
- reflective moments
- memories unconnected with life but appear to recall past events (some believe these are living memories of past lives)

As a personal example, when I write poetry I find it curious that quite often small details appear which I am not conscious of knowing. For example, I wrote of nomads' 'teeth grinding on sand'. When I showed this someone who had travelled extensively with the Bedouin in the Sahara he smiled and said that this was one of the problems they encountered. Whether you consider this guesswork, romanticism or phenomena depends upon your personality – and which of your archetypes is expressing!

Jung was working on matters which were not concrete therefore his research tools were intangible. The title he selected for his autobiography Memories, Dreams and Reflections is a telling indicator of the importance he attached to these areas of mind.

Déjà vu is a particularly interesting phenomenon which scientists are still researching. This may have connections with what is called false memory syndrome, where people are insistent they have experienced something which could not have happened. An interesting movie which demonstrates déjà vu is Groundhog Day.

Remember, Jung's work was decades before scientists discovered genes and genetic inheritance or had access to powerful instruments like brain scanners. If you consider his conclusions in this light, the work is remarkable.

The Behaviourists
Ivan Pavlov [1849 -1936] & John Watson [1878-1958]
Edward Thorndike [1874-1949]
Burrus Skinner [1904 - 1990]

A separate school of thought was developed by the 1930's by Ivan Pavlov who conducted experiments on animal behaviour. Pavlov proved that responses to a stimulus could be changed through his famous experiment with dogs. Pavlov had a bell rung each time his experimental dogs were given food. Before long the dogs started to salivate as soon as they heard the bell, proving the bell and not the food had been the trigger for salivation. His collaborator John Watson continued the work, discovering human behaviour was not naturally inborn but conditioned [changed] through life experience. The two main arguments of Pavlov and Watson are now commonly known as 'nature versus nurture'.

Edward Thorndike and Burrus Skinner enhanced these early behavioural theories. Skinner continued Thorndike's work by placing rats in a maze. The rats were rewarded for going in the right direction or punished by electric shock for going the wrong way. He drew the conclusion that animals and humans learn through reward and punishment. Mental illnesses treated by early behavioural therapy included depressive illness, phobias and addictions to drugs and alcohol.

****

Key Learning
- Morel's Degeneracy Theory –families who practice abuses degenerate over the generations, eventually becoming sterile and dying out
- Phineas Gage and the invention of psycho surgery
- Growing power of Psychiatrists –rise of psychiatry, from unqualified Superintendents of Asylums who were experienced in dealing, pre medications, with patient behaviour
- Meaning of Asylum - place of refuge for patients, not a building
- Freud & Jung – the rise of analysis and the beginning of talking cures
- Behaviourism - that man can learn through reward & punishment

Mental illness is nothing to be ashamed of, but stigma and bias shame us all'
Bill Clinton, former US President

4   MENTAL ILLNESS IN 20TH & 21ST CENTURY

Content:
Lobotomy
Asylums in the 20th Century
Remembering Patient Vulnerability
Token Economy
Encounter Groups
Cognitive Behavioural Therapies
Pioneering Brief Therapy by Milton Erickson
Dr Kathy Sykes – Placebo and Healing
Counselling
Dialectical Behaviour Therapy (DBT)
Medical Treatments: ECT and Drug Therapy
Anti Psychiatric Movement of 60's and 70's:
Virtual Brains - computer simulation

Lobotomy

I mentioned in the last chapter the accident to Phineas Gage, as a result of which Psychiatrists began to seek physical causes for behavioural problems. After the discovery that damage to the frontal lobes lead to changes in personality, scientists began to experiment with a procedure called lobotomy or leucotomy. This was a form of surgery in which the frontal lobes of the brain were detached. It was performed on patients with severe behavioural problems, schizophrenia or untreatable clinical depression, and in some cases appeared to work. The first lobotomy was carried out by Egas Moniz in 1935 who won the 1949 Nobel Prize for his work. As a footnote I gather Egas Moniz was paralysed when he was shot by a patient he had lobotomised. Unfortunately the procedure was taken up by one Walter Freeman who carried out over 2000 operations by sweeping an ice pick under the brow-ridge of his patients. Nearly 50,000 patients underwent operations in the 1950's and ten per cent died. There is no evidence this brutal practice worked and it was discontinued in 1975. Readers might be interested in the movie One Flew Over the Cuckoo's Nest a fictionalised account of a man who had a lobotomy operation with catastrophic consequences.

Asylums in the 20th Century

Asylums had adapted by late 20th century and now provided a home and proper treatment for severely mentally patients unable to live alone or with their families. They also contained surviving patients of the Victorian era, so-called moral defectives who had been put away [historic term] by relatives and spent the remainder of their lives in the Asylum. I met some of the latter whilst doing voluntary work in the 1970's some of them delightful people in their 80's and 90's still with their mental faculties. One patient, branded a social misfit by her parents, had her child taken away and later her husband divorced her. A male patient had stolen a bicycle when he was a teenager and been put away by his embarrassed parents never to return to his community.

Remembering Patient Vulnerability

In the 1990's I met a lovely elderly gentleman (now deceased) who had been found in a dishevelled state after his mother died. He was taken to live in a succession of care homes for blind women until he was placed in the Asylum. He lived there 30 years despite the fact he never had an active mental illness. In his final years he often mourned his missed opportunities, a loss which reminds me of the patients Dr Oliver Sachs movingly describes in 'Awakenings'. One of this man's pet sayings was 'it's a wonderful world', something I expect he was told by a social worker. Please remember the vulnerabilities of institutionalized patients if you come across any. Try to be careful when you present the outside world. To be aware of his loss had cruelly haunted poor Fred. His last few years were spent in the community, shuffling to the shops for foodstuffs which his elderly female housemates made into Victorian high teas. I heard many years later he had been killed in a road traffic accident, a poignant ending to his life.

I remembered being shocked by such stories and this is what first developed my interest in the history of mental illness and my determination to keep the memory of these people alive. Such tragedies seem incredible in the 21st century but they are a very real part of the history of mental illness and should not be forgotten.

Token Economy

Another form of behavioural therapy in vogue in the 1970's was token economy. Patients were rewarded for good behaviour by being given plastic tokens which they could exchange for cigarettes, extra cups of tea and treats like biscuits. Rather animalistic yet human nature always triumphs; what the psychologists on the Ward I worked on might not have realized was the black economy in tokens late at night.

Encounter Groups

Encounter groups were developed by Carl Rogers with the aim of improving human potential. Group members were encouraged to discuss their deepest feelings with other members. These groups later became infamous for the potential to cause psychological damage through less than careful group leaders. This therapy is now discredited.

Cognitive Behavioural Therapies

Cognitive (cognitive = to recognise) therapists came to believe that people who consistently experienced frustrations, anxieties and emotional problems had faulty thinking patterns. They attributed negative thinking patterns to poor and repeated behaviour patterns, which developed as a result of negative life experiences. By recognizing, challenging and changing this dysfunctional thinking, associated negative emotions and behaviour could be changed. Behavioural and cognitive therapy were combined into cognitive-behavioural therapy, which remains popular.

Pioneering Brief Therapy by Milton Erickson

In the 1970's Erickson (an American Psychiatrist) pioneered a quirky method which rapidly had patients flocking to his clinics. During his early life, Erickson developed polio and was confined to his bed. Bored, Erickson started observing visitors, noting their body language. Over many years he became expert at observing what he called his patient's personal map of the world. Erickson watched his young siblings from the time they crawled to when they first walked. From these observations he taught himself to walk from scratch. Erickson came to the conclusion that everyone has a key to resolving their own problems and the work of the therapist is to help them apply these strategies to their current problems.

Erickson initially advocated auto-hypnosis whereby the patient, in a very relaxed state, could imagine themselves free of their problem and describe how life would be without it. From that starting point Erickson set patients tasks to enhance the healing effect.

Erickson was interested in the symbolism of language. He learned to talk to patients using their symbolic language (metaphors). The crux of his method was establishing the problem from the patient's point of view and at the same time enhancing the therapeutic relationship.

Dr Kathy Sykes – Placebo and Healing

The therapeutic relationship is often undervalued but is recognised as a known phenomenon with great importance in healing. A Channel 4 programme by Dr Kathy Sykes found evidence that a therapeutic relationship (placebo effect) does make a difference. During the programme CAT scans were shown of patient's pain centres. During healing sessions, these pain centres visibly diminished in size.

Counselling

There are hundreds of types of talking therapy and new schools of thought spring up all the time. Freud and Jung, the roots of this vast tree, might be very surprised if they could see the fruits of their theories. Some schools favour individual counselling, others within groups; some believe the dynamic of relationship is paramount whilst others believe social interaction is the only way of maintaining mental health. Some schools use problem solving whilst analytical types seek insight as a key to change. There is a grey area between counselling and psychotherapy which are often interchangeable. The common denominator is that talking is the major tool of therapy unlike medical practitioners who use the tools of surgery, medication and techniques like ECT.

Dialectical Behaviour Therapy (DBT)

Dialectical behaviour therapy (DBT) was developed by American Psychologist Marsha Lineham for patients with personality disorders. Dialectical means at either end. The name reflects both ends of the high emotional states experienced by people with personality disorders. DBT aims to pull the extremes together so the patient learns neither to hide nor overtly express feelings but make him or herself reasonably understood, to become less critical and at the same time less self critical.

In DBT the relationship between therapist and patient has to be cooperative as they are dealing with the delicate area of patient belief. DBT develops positive behaviours in individual situations, promotes self understanding and offers reward through praise. Patients who undergo DBT are very likely to have felt criticized most of their lives. DBT aims to build on success and spread change through all unproductive behaviours.

Medical Treatments: ECT and Drug Therapy

I have already mentioned early experiments by the Romans with electric eels and attempts to give shocks to Asylum patients using eels. These historic systems were replaced with electric currents after the discovery of electricity by Franklin and later Edison. Modern ECT was used for treating shell-shocked soldiers and depressive illness with some success.

After the 1950's a drug called lithium was used to treat mania and manic depressive psychosis. Early anti-psychotic drugs such as Largactil were known as liquid coshes because they made patients lethargic. In the 1960's tranquillisers Librium and Valium were prescribed to generations of women for nervous disorders until being withdrawn from general use when they were found addictive.

Medication rather than psychological therapies was at its height throughout these decades until the 1980's and the rise of Prozac. Heralded as a wonder drug and cure for depression this class of drugs [called SSRI's –

see the 2nd book of this series] were marked as potentially causal in suicide.

Medication is not a panacea, even when evidence based. You have to treat the patient as Hippocrates and many of his successors advocated. The tide is turning with complementary and brief [talking] therapies gaining popularity as the 21st century penchant for open-talk about mental health gains momentum and psychiatry declines in favour of more natural cures.

Anti Psychiatric Movement of 60's and 70's:

Thomas Szaz, R. D. Laing : *'In psychiatry, we use one set of laws to explain sane behaviour, which we attribute to reasons (choices) and another set of laws to explain insane behaviour, which we attribute to causes (diseases).'* Thomas Szaz 2001.

Psychiatrists Szaz and Laing held the controversial view that mental illness did not exist but was a construct of society. Laing considered the symptoms of madness to be insights that is psychoses held symbolic [metaphorical] meaning. It is easier to explain this by example so I will offer you one of my own experiences.

Several months prior to a psychosis I dreamt I was riding a motorbike when the fuel tank catch slipped open and the top of the tank reared in front of me. I calmly got off the bike and then the fuel tank burst into flames. This dream has overtones of sexuality and danger. At the time of this dream my marriage was breaking up and I was virtually homeless and penniless. The dream indicated I would recover from psychosis [calm feeling] which was indeed what occurred. The symbolism of a motorbike is appropriate; my interests in historic machinery, archaeology and being born in an industrial town. If you are interested in dream analysis try C G Jung's book Man and His Symbols.

The anti-psychiatric movement grew as service users (people who use mental health services), frustrated with bad side effects of drugs and lack of other effective treatments sought other answers. The anti-psychiatry books by Szaz, Laing and their followers make interesting reading, especially when seen in the light of 21st century preference for talking or complementary therapies rather than medication.

Virtual Brains - computer simulation

Real hope for rapid progress in understanding mental illness has come about through attempts to build computer-simulated (virtual) human brains. This will stimulate faster results for example on research of faulty genes responsible for serious illness such as schizophrenia. Such research would normally take decades but thanks to computers this is speeded up. Perhaps we are nearing the time when mental illness becomes a thing of the past like polio. I would love to be alive to see this happen.

****

Key Learning:
- Lobotomy in movies - One Flew Over the Cuckoo's Nest - a fictional account of man undergoing lobotomy with catastrophic consequences.
- Patient vulnerability - vulnerabilities of institutionalized patients. Try to be careful when you present the outside world to such patients.
- Medication not always helpful - medication is not a panacea. Treat the patient, as Hippocrates advocated.
- Computers and the mind - knowledge is building at a fantastic rate.

Figure 11 Electro-Convulsive Therapy & Medication

ELECTRO-CONVULSIVE THERAPY & DRUG THERAPY:
Two methods of restoring 'balance' in brain chemistry

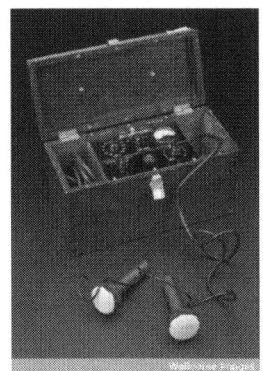

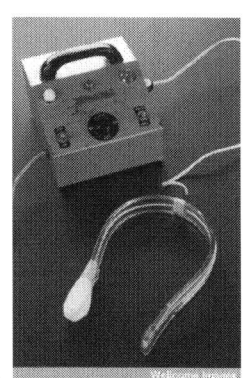

ECT control box - permission
Wellcome Picture Library

ECT
Patients are given sedatives & muscle relaxant. Small electrodes are attached to each side of the skull and an electric current discharged into the brain. The attending Psychiatrist controls the strength & timing of the current.

Drug Therapy
Drugs are given orally or by injection.

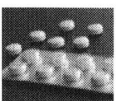

Anti depressants are synthesised versions of the naturally occurring brain chemicals, Dopamine, Noradrenaline and Serotonin. These chemicals are considered responsible for regulating mood.

'Not nice.. the mattress is mouldy, the food bland.. most of my day is spent looking out a window waiting for a Doctor to arrive.'
Personal experience - NHS Psychiatric Hospital

5 PSYCHIATRIC HOSPITALS, COMMUNITY CARE

Content:
NHS & Community Act
Sale / Disposal of Asylum Buildings
Re-housing for Mental Patients
New Build Psychiatric Hospitals & Centres
Rehabilitation Units
Multi Disciplinary Professional Teams
Inter-Team Rivalries and Varying Quality of Leadership
Outreach Care
Where Next?

NHS & Community Act

In the 1990's, the NHS & Community Act sent mental patients to live in the community in a cosy hope their fellow humans would help re-integrate them into community life. Treatment outside hospital had become possible because of the advent of drugs. Most patients no longer required overseeing or restraint and it seemed the days of the bins (historic term 'looney bins') were over. Whether rightly or wrongly, there was a lot of fear in the community about this measure. Many people had experienced mental patients only through reading the sensationalist newspaper headlines, such as I describe in the chapters on social exclusion. This lack of education had been vastly under estimated and early patient settlements were to pay the price. Some patients found themselves lonely and isolated, some were threatened by local vigilantes, though it was true the more fortunate were welcomed by their new neighbours.

Sale / Disposal of Asylum Buildings

There remained a kind of irony, of former crumbling Asylum buildings now purchased by property developers and refurbished into expensive homes for the middle classes. Unlike other historic buildings where origins and history are proudly displayed on blue plaques or detailed signage, all links to former Asylum were are often removed. St John's Hospital, where I worked, had to be pulled down when thieves stole the lead off the roof and the rain ruined what was left of the buildings, including the listed chapel.

NHS engineers struggled for decades to maintain Victorian buildings with cranky heating systems, draughty windows, peeling paint and stonework. As mental patients were moved into not-so-sexy social housing, the rich and educated new owners moved into newly refurbished luxury flats and water-tower penthouses which developers carved out of the former Asylum buildings. This was an example of how the NHS failed to protect assets, first in removing security guards 'because they were too expensive', second in failing to protect listed buildings, then selling their property portfolio for a fraction of the true value.

Re-housing for Mental Patients

At the same time, mental patients were not provided with sufficient social support. Many were moved into isolated flats, with weekly visits from staff but no other means, after decades of institutionalization. It was perhaps underestimated, because Managers did not consider this re-housing from the patients point of view – no friends, little money and no relatives make for social isolation, then as now. The best choice were group homes, with several patients living together, sometimes former friends from the asylum. And was it good or bad, how one group home was sited next door to a small police station whose officers did not realize who was next door.

No education for the community was a large error. And hopefully in the future communities will not whitewash large chunks of what they consider 'distasteful' history.

Now I re-write this in 2015 there is a resurgence in family history, with programmes such as Who Do You Think You Are bringing many sad stories of wasted lives to the fore. The last of the patients is long dead, but their memory must live on, for all they suffered. I hope those who have any mementoes or memories to inform their local Records Office and give any information or images. This period of history should never be lost to time.

New Build Psychiatric Hospitals & Centres

An average new-build small scale psychiatric hospital might comprise one or two permanent wards, day hospital and teaching facilities. These hospitals were built in major towns and lacked large open spaces and specialist buildings [chapels, laundries etc] which made Asylums into mini towns. The grounds of these buildings, being sited within towns, were small. Very little space for patients to relax, let off steam or allow staff a pleasant lunch hour. Those sited within earlier Asylum buildings would fare better. The Reception area was common to seriously mentally ill and day patients. This lead to consternation among day patients, unused to seeing seriously ill patients. Was this a planning faux pas or was it meant to create a de-stigmatizing environment? What do you think?

Figure 12   St John's Hospital, Stone, Near Aylesbury

Chapel

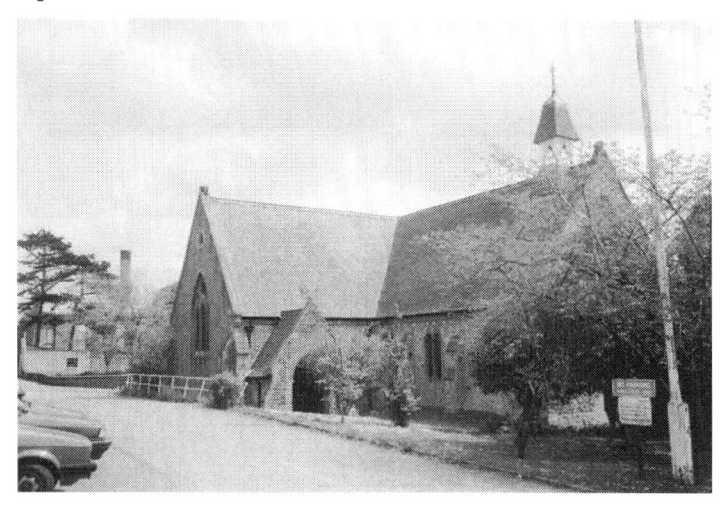

Main Entrance and Water Tower

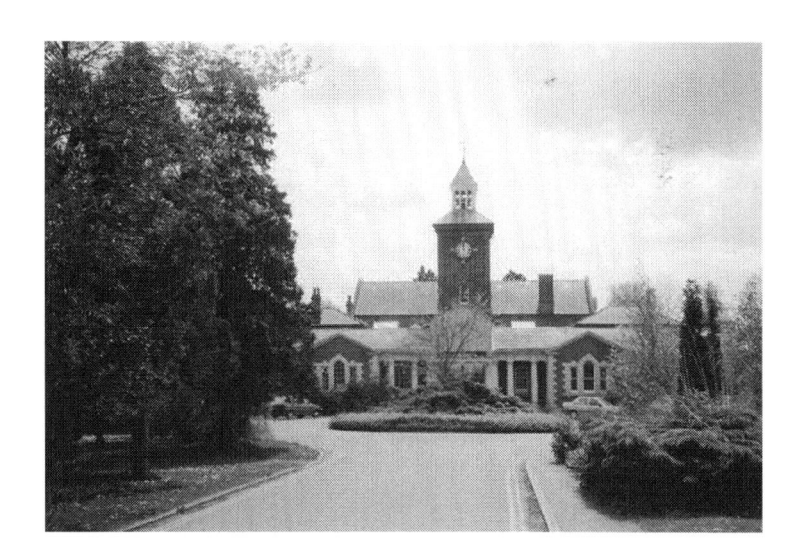

Small consulting rooms, on the lines of those in private healthcare, housed therapists who treated day patients. The rooms were small, housing a coffee table, couple of chairs and maybe a filing cabinet. Even these were larger than a room I once worked in within Primary Care which was less than 6' square; marginally larger than a rabbit hutch and about as well equipped with overflowing bins left by a Practice Manager who disapproved of counselling and liked staff to know it.

Team rooms where the multi-disciplinary teams worked were basic, with a central space for the team to gather and some hot desks around the edges. Hot-desking, where employees share desks on a first-come first-served basis, was not favoured and lead to many rumbles.

Wards for short-stay relapses were small and few in number. You might count the number of patients on two hands. Some psychiatric hospitals had larger wards and were complete treatment centres.

Larger new build psychiatric hospitals, such as the one I had the bad luck to stay in, would house short-term patients. These had more facilities such as art therapy rooms, dining rooms and consulting rooms. However, these were smaller than the range found in Asylums and catered for fewer patients. Lack of space was a continuing issue and lead to conflicts.

Each Psychiatric Hospital would not only deal with long-term (chronic) patients but also with day patients. Day-case patients were referrals from Primary Care (GP surgeries) and might typically not have active mental illness but emotional or behavioural problems, mainly stress. These patients were colloquially referred to as 'the worried well'.

Rehabilitation Units

Very few patients would be admitted to Psychiatric Hospitals for long stay, in fact the new regime was only meant for short admittances for relapse. Outpatient care was only possible for those with enduring mental illness because of effective medications and readily-available therapy. Rehabilitation Units were built as small scale longer term home units for small groups of seriously ill patients under rehabilitation. Eventually, they too would be re-integrated in the community. Rehab Units were a halfway house between hospital and living in the community. It is not easy living with major mental illness with the noise, strangeness and confusion of community life, still less if that community is dysfunctional.

In the Unit I visited, the Manager had enabled community members with little or no experience of mental patients to be introduced to their new neighbours in a gradual way, by providing social opportunities such as Fetes and talks about the Unit. Patients were not 'on show', but given tasks such as running stalls, which enabled them to grow their social skills. They were encourages to sign on and attend local adult education classes, using every aspect from planning buses to finding classes, to improve confidence.

figure 13 Victorian Asylum Patients

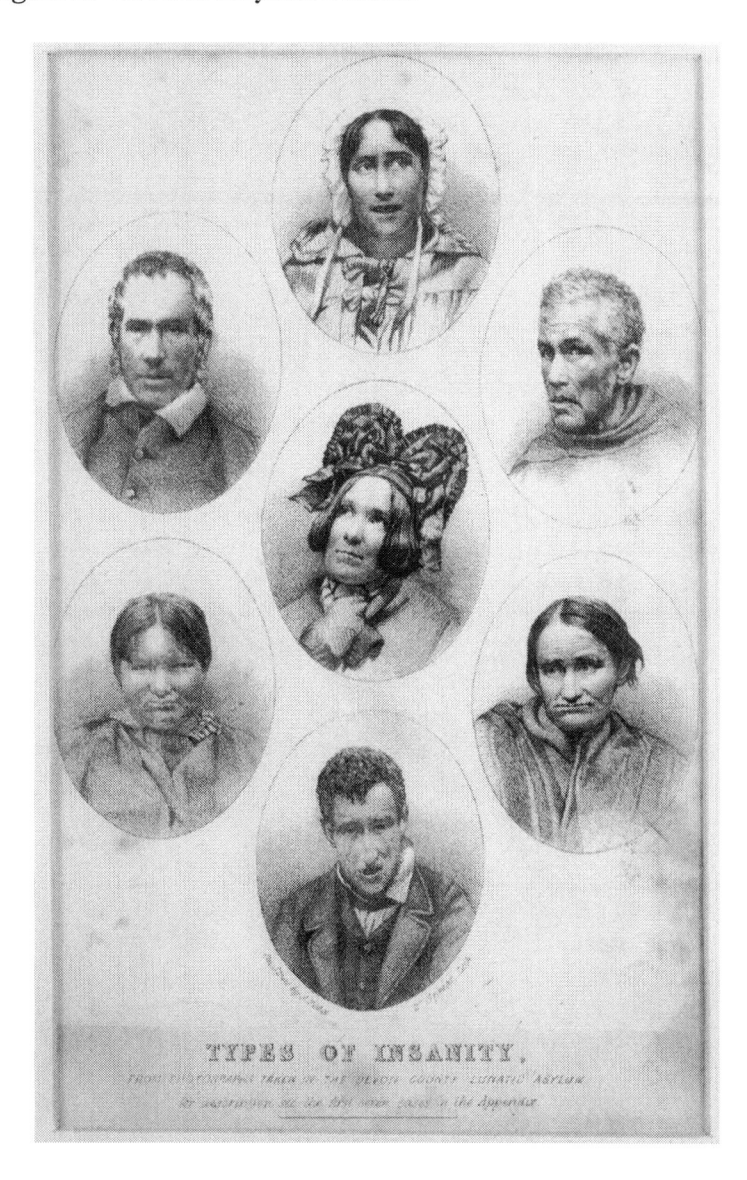

Multi Disciplinary Professional Teams

Within Psychiatric Hospitals (or Centres as they were sometimes called) staff worked in mixed discipline mental health teams, comprising psychiatry, psychology, occupational therapy, social work, mental nursing and rehabilitation. Generally, Psychiatrists took the lead role, much to the chagrin of some of the Nurses.

Inter-Team Rivalries and Varying Quality of Leadership

As in any team, there was jockeying for position, with overlaps between roles causing friction and, sadly, bullying going on. Some teams were better lead and organized. This was in fact my first experience of being bullied at work. I am unsure if these teams were educated about groups and group behaviour, but it was a sad lack in my team. If this is so in yours, perhaps time to redress?

My first experience had a 'nice' Nurse who nevertheless was a poor leader and allowed himself to be bullied by a rather unpleasant female nurse (the same one who bullied me). Not quite accepted by the medics, being a new profession themselves, Mental Nurses made new professionals unwelcome. I expect this cycle will repeat until new grade Graduate Mental Health Workers come on board.

Individuals met weekly to take on patients referred by Primary Care (GP surgeries) and discuss continuing care for longer term patients. Patients (long term or day cases) would be seen either at the Hospital or Centre or at home if that was more convenient for them. It was the beginning of a true community care programme.

Outreach Care

As well as the Psychiatric Hospital or centre-based Community Mental Health Teams there were other teams of professionals providing care for different circumstances:

- Assertive Outreach (for chronically mentally ill patients)
- Emergency Duty Teams (for emergency treatments)
- Early Intervention For Psychosis Team
- Samaritans (voluntary service charity for the suicidal)

There were of links with Primary Care (GP surgeries) for patients with frequent relapse patterns who might otherwise fall out of the care network. Gaps between services were a major reason for seriously-ill psychiatric patients not having medication monitored and going on to commit serious criminal offences as a result of delusions. These were the cases which caused the sensationalist headlines and resulted in a great deal of misunderstandings about mental illness.

figure 14 St John's Hospital – Montage

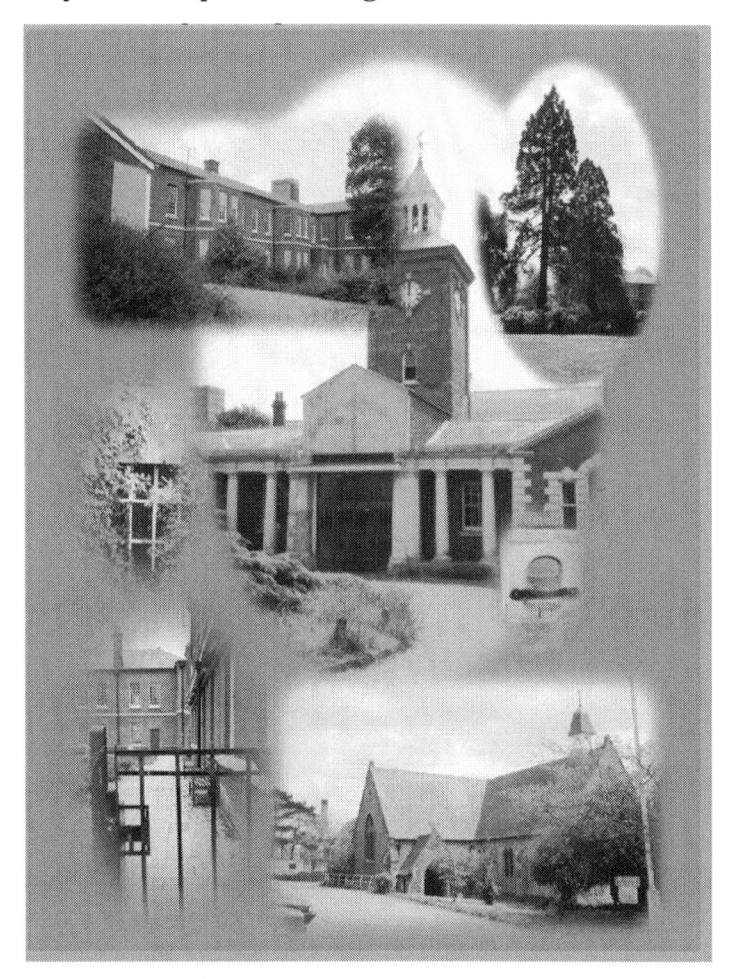

Where Next?

There were plans for a complete overhaul to the service which involved a major re-structuring of the mental health work force. A new Mental Health Degree course was introduced in 2000, with the aim of creating a new breed of Graduate Mental Health Workers. This was to be the core course with further professional training (including medical) branching off from this. What a good idea you might think but unfortunately this hit the old guard in the pants; medics, nurses, psychologists and therapists who feared their imminent demise. This again was an error of judgement – lack of education to long-standing staff, leading to bullying as it inevitably will.

****

Key Learning

- Care in the Community Act – patients treated in the community, living in flats and adapted homes. Good or bad idea?
- lack of education –community unprepared for re-siting of mentally ill patients into their community
- Reception Areas separation zones? Separation between the 'worried well' and patients with enduring mental illness, to prevent former being subjected to bizarre behaviours? What do you think?
- Interdisciplinary teams – were they educated in group behaviour to prevent overlap of professions and rivalries?
- Bullying –nipped in the bud when there is a common training; parity without compromising ambition?
- Graduate Mental Health Workers – new training but a threat to the old guard? How might this have been prevented?

> '..callous belief that the insane do not suffer and that any problems they may express are bound to be 'imaginary'.
> Roy Porter in Madness, A Brief History

6   MENTAL HEALTH ACT 1983

Content
Definitions of Professionals in the 1983 Act
Sections of the 1983 Act
Applications for Sections
Section 2 – Admission for Assessment
Section 3 – Admission for Treatment
Section 4 – Emergency admission
Section 20 – Renewal (of a Section)
Section 23 – Discharge
Sections 57 Consent to Treatment
Section 58 Consent (with 2nd opinion)
Section 93 Management of Financial Affairs
Section 134 – Withholding of Correspondence
Section 135 – Power to Enter (Private) premises
Section 136 – Removal from Public Places
Epilogue

The stated aim of the Mental Health Act 1983 is 'the reception, care and treatment of mentally disordered patients, the management of their property and other related matters'. This is the legal machinery by which those considered a danger to themselves or the public can be forcibly treated.

The Act is divided into sections, which is the origin of the term sectioning as used to describe how someone is taken into care '(s)he was sectioned'.

Definitions of Professionals in the 1983 Act
The Act specifies responsibilities of mental health workers:
- Approved Social Worker (ASW) special Social Workers trained in Mental Health Act law
- Mental Health Review Tribunal (MHRT) professional and non professional people appointed by the Lord Chancellor
- Nearest Relative - close relative of the patient e.g. spouse, partner, parent who is over 18
- Responsible Medical Officer (RMO) – the Doctor or Psychiatrist responsible for the medical care of the patient

Sections of the 1983 Act

On being sectioned, your letters might be opened. You are not allowed to walk alone in the grounds of the hospital. Once a patient has been detained in psychiatric hospital for a long period of time there is a danger of institutionalization. After weeks or months being cared for, people lose the will and the social skills needed to live outside the confines of a hospital, indeed becomes a frightening process. We call this institutionalization.

Applications for Sections

Applications have to be made for all sections of the 1983 Act. These are formal papers which legally enable someone to be admitted to Hospital for treatment even if they do not wish to go. Applications are made by an Approved Social Worker or qualified Doctors or Psychiatrists.

Section 2 – Admission for Assessment

This section is used for:
- persons not admitted before
- existing patients of mental health service
- on application from 2 medical recommendations
- detention for up to 28 days
- grounds for sectioning–a severe mental disorder which needs hospital assessment and it is in his/her safety or safety of the public

Two doctors may detain for 28 days under this section. This is a long time to be in a psychiatric hospital, especially if it is the first time. Imagine yourself sectioned. Can you imagine how anxiety-provoking this might be? How would you cope living 28 days with severely mentally ill people if you're unused to bizarre behaviour or strong expressed emotion? Would family and friends visit or would they be too embarrassed?

Section 3 – Admission for Treatment

Admission applications are signed by 2 medical referees. The patient can be admitted for up to six months. This application can be renewed after six months and then annually. There are only 2 grounds for admission:
- patient safety
- protection of the public

Relatives can protest about admission but have to give reasonable grounds for refusal. They were highly unlikely to be successful because professionals made decisions using their knowledge of the law.

Section 4 – Emergency admission

Emergency admission for treatment can be made by a Doctor, and a patient can be admitted up to 72 hours (3 days) for assessment. If the Doctor is tired or does not know the patient, God help them if he has to make a decision in a hurry. The patient about to be admitted might be of different culture, or naturally lively or aggressive, which might colour the doctor's opinion.

Section 20 – Renewal (of a Section)

This allows renewal of sections for 6 months then further periods of one year. The Doctor has to prove the patient will improve or not deteriorate if treatment is given and that this is in the best interests of the patient or public or both. Mental Health Managers have to review the patient. These people are members of the Mental Health Trust Board with varying degrees of experience in mental health.

Imagine how a new patient might be affected if for the first time they are living in the company of seriously ill mental patients.

Section 23 – Discharge

When the patient is fit to be discharged their nearest relative can request early discharge. Tribunals can overrule this request if the patient is considered dangerous. If the patient wishes to remain in hospital (by no means uncommon) the Tribunal will make that decision too.

The danger is misinterpretation of symptoms. In a recent report I read of someone described as psychotic because they entered a room then left in a hurry. Perhaps they needed the toilet or maybe they were autistic? It is easy for beginners to over-interpret and look for signs of illness. This is the halo effect; if you are convinced someone is ill, you are likely to see symptoms. It is easy to misinterpret. As an analogy, if you were told someone had a cold and they sneezed that might prove they had a cold, because that is what you were expecting. What if they were allergic to dust.

Sections 57 Consent to Treatment

Section 57 is about consent to treatment with psycho (brain) surgery or hormonal implants for patients who have given voluntary consent. The proposed surgery must be proven to cure or alleviate the condition and 3 medical professionals must confirm the patient understands the nature of the treatment they are to undergo. Psycho surgery includes lobotomy, which is now rarely performed. It involves detaching the frontal lobes of the brain to modify behaviour. In the past this surgery had devastating effects on the patient's intellect and mood. It is irreversible.

Surgery is dangerous and it has to be ascertained that patients are aware of the implications. Danger to the public is a powerful consideration but mental health charities are worried these powers will impede human rights.

Section 58 Consent (with 2nd opinion)

This section is consent to treatment by medication or ECT (electro convulsive therapy) for patients who understand what the treatment involves but have NOT given permission for treatment.

In these cases the Mental Health Act Commission appoint a 2nd opinion Doctor who has to agree that treatment will be beneficial. ECT is highly regulated and can only be performed in certain circumstances. ECT is dangerous and Psychiatrists do not know how or even if, it will work.

The easiest way to learn about these treatments is to watch 2 movies: 'A Beautiful Mind' for early ECT treatment; 'One Flew over the Cuckoo's Nest' for worst-case scenario lobotomy.

Section 93 Management of Financial Affairs

The Court of Protection can give a relative or professional Power of Attorney over the financial affairs of a sectioned patient that is they are given legal permission to manage that person's finances. The person appointed has to keep financial records, report to the Court and are required to act in the best interest of the patient. This is a controversial section as you might imagine.

Section 134 – Withholding of Correspondence

If a patient is likely to send offensive or dangerous material by post the Courts have the right to issue orders that any post sent out can be withheld (except curiously for mail sent to an MP) and incoming mail vetted.

Manic patients sometimes send sexually explicit letters that embarrass the recipient (and the patient, when they recover). Patients under delusions can send threatening material or receive goods they intend to use for malicious purposes; guns, knives or bombs. Although these are valid reasons for vetting and withholding mail under extreme circumstances, such laws have to be applied without unnecessarily curtailing civil liberty. Freedom to live does not confer license to act in such a way that others suffer.

Section 135 – Power to Enter (Private) premises

If someone is hiding in private premises or their own home and it is believed they are mentally ill, Police Officers can obtain a warrant from a Justice of the Peace to forcibly enter the premises. In most sectioning cases, relatives have called Social Services or the police, perhaps after suffering for many weeks.

I have seen extreme suffering in some cases, for example the elderly parents of a friend whose daughter was sectioned for mania every few years.

The sectioning would often be weeks after she had become high, leaving them in an anxious state, unable to sleep for fear of what she might do. It is difficult, because Social Workers can be reluctant to section, knowing the social consequences. A Social Worker with an ASW qualification and a Doctor must be present at the time of entry. The potential patient can be taken to a place of safety where they can be kept for up to 72 hours (3 days).

Sectioning can be frightening. Imagine your loved one carried screaming or crying from the house by burly police officers with neighbours gawping. It is not pleasant. Imagine you are mentally ill with flashes of awareness. How do you cope when you realize you have been ejected from your home, a relative has been put in charge of your finances and your letters withheld.

Section 136 – Removal from Public Places

A police officer can remove anyone from a public area for mental health assessment and keep them in a place of safety for up to 72 hours (3 days). Police officers are not trained mental health workers although some Health Authorities provide courses. This lack of knowledge can lead to misunderstandings. Section 136 is controversial, particularly in multi cultural communities with many different lifestyles and social norms. Here are a couple of examples:

- Black youths generally do not give eye contact; it is not considered respectful in their culture. Police have been known to misinterpret this as being belligerent.
- In spiritualist cultures seeing visions is normal. Such visions have been misinterpreted as psychotic symptoms.

I strongly advise new Mental Health Workers in multi cultural urban areas to bone up on cultural issues.

Epilogue

I hope you have a clearer idea of some of the issues involved in developing and interpreting mental health law. There are considerations which depend upon which hat you are wearing; mental health worker, police, patient or mental health charity worker. This is why it is good to role play and become familiar with different scenarios.

Try this exercise with colleagues. Set an imaginary case history which involves someone being sectioned. Each participant selects a role from the list below, and afterwards you can discuss findings:

- Carer
- Patient
- Mental Health Worker
- ASW Social Worker

- Police[wo]man
- Neighbour
- Postal Worker
- Government Minister
- Journalist

Learn to consider the Mental Health Act from many points of view, not just the role you are employed in. This will give you a rounded view and help you understand the patient better.

****

Key Learning
- How It Feels to be Sectioned - Imagine yourself, a friend or relative being sectioned. Clinicians are making decisions which have serious consequences for your future.
- How would you cope living 28 days in the presence of severely mentally ill people if you're unused to bizarre behaviour?
- Would family and friends visit or would they be too embarrassed?
- Over-interpretation of Symptoms- As an analogy if you were told someone had a cold and they sneezed that might 'prove' they had a cold, because it is what you are expecting – but it might be hay fever.
- ECT & Psychosurgery - watch 2 movies: 'A Beautiful Mind' for early ECT treatment; 'One Flew over the Cuckoo's Nest' for worst-case scenario lobotomy.
- Freedom v License - Freedom does not automatically confer license to act in such a way that someone else suffers.
- Insight During Illness - Imagine you are mentally ill but with flashes of awareness. How do you cope when you realize you have been ejected from your home, a relative has been put in charge of your finances and your letters are withheld.
- Look at the Act from Many Points of View - not just the role you are employed in. This will give you a rounded view of the difficulties involved and help you understand the patient.

"The Bill..aims to [help] early .. so fewer people reach crisis level."
Rosie Winterton (Minister for Health)

7 PROPOSED MENTAL HEALTH BILL 2004

This chapter contains:
Why New Legislation
Proposed 2004 Bill – Flowchart
Fears about Proposed 2004 Bill
Summary of Mind's Proposals for a New Act
Government's Response to Public Questions
Updates on Mental Health Law, 2005 & 2007

The proposed Mental Health Bill 2004 has been discarded following protest by individuals and mental health charities. However, as a piece of mental health history it is important for students to understand the process. I have extracted bare facts from a variety of sources. Consider the aspects of law:

- moral: care for patient (human rights) and safety of public
- in the light of modern medication & community care
- £Ms committed to treat & reduce stigma

Try to put yourself in the roles from the previous chapter, because this will help understand the law from different angles:
- Carer
- Patient
- Mental Health Worker
- ASW Social Worker
- Police[wo]man
- Neighbour
- Postal Worker
- Government Minister
- Journalist

This exercise will give a rounded view. I remember how many of the Social Workers and Mental Nurses I worked with a decade ago held strong, sometimes opposing, views on mental health law. I do not believe they were practicing the multi-faceted thinking of rounded mental health workers. Do pat yourself on the back if you take the time and trouble to do these exercises!

Why New Legislation

Community care and effective medication changed the environment where Mental Health Act 1983 was operating. There are more services for patients with serious mental illnesses outside hospital and better medication. However, civil liberties remain paramount and European Law has to be taken into account. These necessaries must be balanced with consideration for public anxiety, albeit the number of patients with serious personality disorders is minimal.

The 2004 Bill was aimed 'improv[ing] the provision of mental health services and mak[ing] them more focused on the needs of the individual' (Department of Health). The original proposals changed a great deal during readings as a result of many comments expressed by mental health charities and members of the public, invited to comment via the Government website. Mental health charities feared the erosion of civil liberties among ex-patients who were not a danger to the public. Mind kindly provided me with a summary of these comments and I append this at the end of the chapter.

The 1983 Act was unclear, for example the reason for detention on grounds of patient safety read 'for the health or safety of the patient'. This was open to wide interpretation. The new Bill aimed for new structures, which would be: 'for the protection of the patient from suicide or serious self-harm or serious neglect by him of his health or safety' (extract from Mental Health Bill 2004).

There were 3 parts to the proposed Bill. The first explained the provisions. Part two explained civil procedures. Part three considered the links with the criminal justice system. The latter was important, because many people felt mentally ill patients should not be imprisoned or be treated in prisons, merely because there was nowhere else for them to be treated. The Government's wanted the Bill to: 'define.. clear and fair procedures for assessment and treatment [and a] new Tribunal system that will authorise use of formal powers beyond the initial assessment of the patient.'

The Government were determined to clarify the reasons for someone to be detained, having burned their fingers on the last writing of the Act.

Figure 15 Proposed 2004 Bill Flowchart

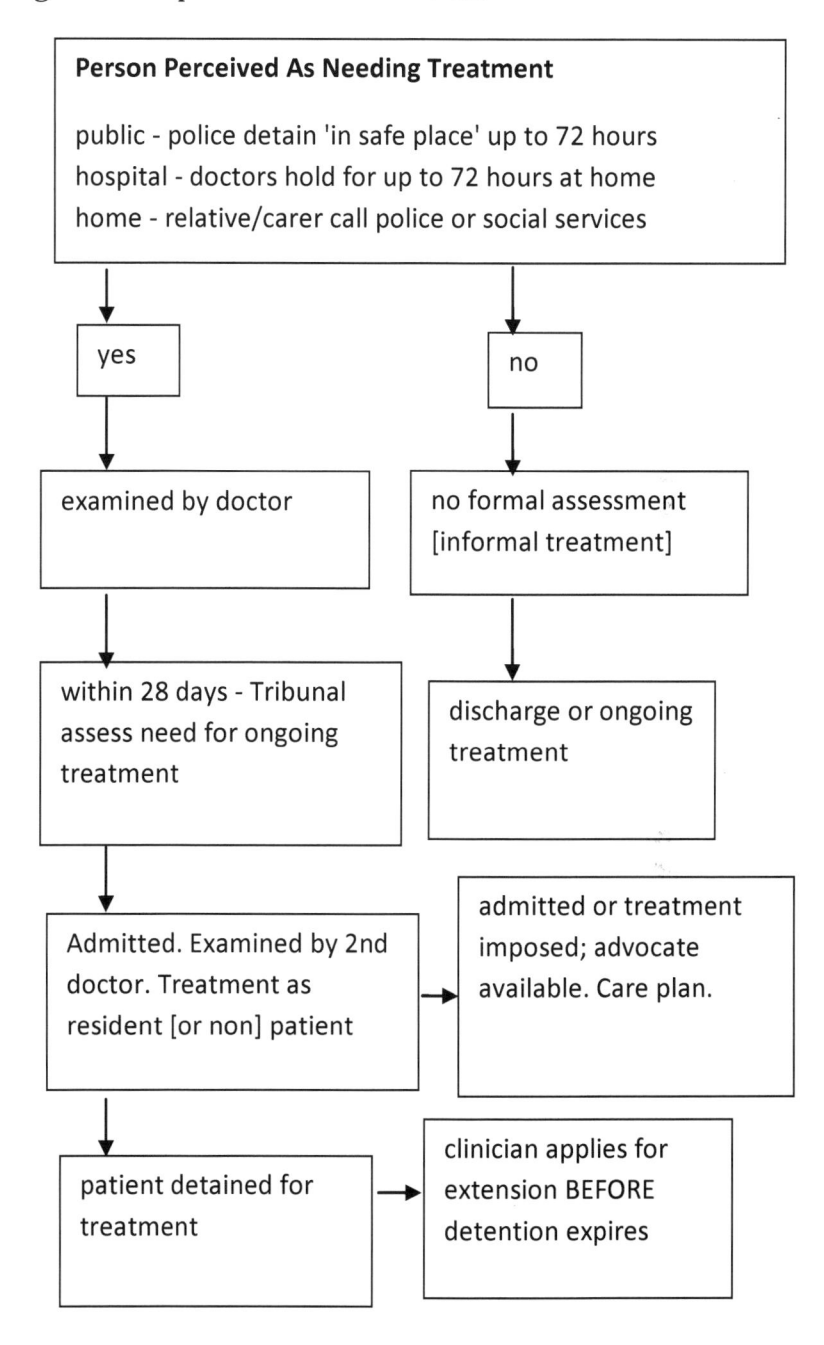

Person Perceived As Needing Treatment

public - police detain 'in safe place' up to 72 hours
hospital - doctors hold for up to 72 hours at home
home - relative/carer call police or social services

- yes → examined by doctor → within 28 days - Tribunal assess need for ongoing treatment → Admitted. Examined by 2nd doctor. Treatment as resident [or non] patient → admitted or treatment imposed; advocate available. Care plan.
  → patient detained for treatment → clinician applies for extension BEFORE detention expires

- no → no formal assessment [informal treatment] → discharge or ongoing treatment

The Bill called for a potential patient to be suffering: 'a mental disorder of such a nature or degree as to warrant the provision of treatment under the supervision of a specialist doctor or senior mental health practitioner.' Treatment had to meet one or of the following conditions:

- protection of the patient from suicide serious self-harm
- serious neglect of their health or safety
- protection of others
- treatment cannot be provided unless powers in the Bill are used
- treatment must be available

Fears about Proposed 2004 Bill

One of the major fears was that the proposed Bill appeared as a means of controlling people considered a danger to society and that they would be subject to forcible treatment – which opposes human rights. Further, mental health charities feared powers might be used to detain people who were not mentally ill but unconventional or eccentric. This might seem far-fetched unless you have been involved in borderline cases. With the added risk of a lengthy confinement, as sections can be extended for long periods, you might begin to appreciate the broad reach of these laws.

Being sectioned is not only loss of liberty but the start of cataclysmic changes in relationships, social life and career, to say nothing of stigmatization. These are considerations which adversely affect people's lives. Sectioning can result in severe mental scarring with lasting effects on personality. Clinicians had fears about the Bill. They feared being forced to give patients treatment in the community and their role would be one of policing. This was not the role they trained for. They also feared Tribunals would be given a more powerful role to detain patients without professional consultation. The Proposed 2004 Bill Flowchart on the previous page was prepared from the Department of Health's initial publication about the Bill.

Quite a bit of controversy as you can see and perhaps it is no wonder the exasperated Government, after all the work, abandoned the Bill. Their main stance had always been protection of the public with patient safety. Too many headlines about psychotic killers which blamed Ministers had taken their political toll.

It is useful to role play, with your peers, a scenario under which potential patient risk is balanced with human rights.

Summary of Mind's Proposals for a New Act

The following list was kindly provided by a member of the media team for Mind (a major mental health charity). I quote it in full as requested:

- 'that general principles should be on the face of the Act
- that the Code of Practice should have mandatory status
- that there should be narrower conditions for the exercise of compulsory powers – in particular removing the possibility of using compulsory powers on people with full decision-making capacity and retaining a test of therapeutic benefit.
- no compulsion in the community
- improved safeguards for advocates & nominated persons
- statutory recognition of the role of advance statements
- a reconstitution of the tribunal to include a role for non-medical members and service users
- an improved duty to provide aftercare
- removal of police power to enter private premises without a warrant
- the right of accused persons to the same safeguards (nominated person, Tribunal) as for civil patients
- a complete prohibition on the administration of ECT on all patients who have capacity and who have refused treatment, and (except for saving life) on all patients without capacity.
- legally binding safeguards to protect people from potentially hazardous practices, including a specific requirement that doses above British National Formulary [the manual which limits the dosage of medications] limits should not be given without informed consent.'

The Government's Response to Public Questions

The Government did not want to make the same errors they had in the Mental Health Act 1983. Realizing public confidence had been damaged they knew they needed to tread a fine line between appeasing the public and not enraging those who worked in mental health services. Controversially, they opened the possibility to mental health professionals other than Social Workers to take statutory roles, offering specialist training, a move guaranteed to make fur fly.

On Detention

An innovative part of the Bill allowed potential patients who were not considered a risk to receive voluntary treatment in the community. This right was to be extended to existing patients and not those new to the services. It was made clear that dangerous patients would not have the choice of voluntary community treatment and Tribunals would be given power to detain. At the same time families were reassured their loved ones would have access to appeal. Patients who required services would be offered advocacy. On the other hand, it was stressed that no one could be

detained, unless:
- they had a recognized mental disorder
- were a threat to the public
- were suicidal
- were likely to commit self harm or neglect themselves
- there was a suitable treatment source already available

On Treatment

The proposal was not for home treatment but at specialist outpatient clinics. Any patient failing to attend the designated clinic would be required to become a resident patient. The same deal was to be extended to forensic patients who were not considered a danger to the community.

In order to clear the fuzzy line between criminality and mental illness (the so-called mad or bad debate) Courts would be given enhanced powers to make decisions about treatment; in the case of minor offenders, they would be offered a mental health order instead of going to prison.

How Patients Benefit from the Bill

So many patients had slipped the net over the years that the Government were determined to take measures to close gaps between services. It was the intention to give everyone a right to advocacy and representation and limit the time patients could be detained without a decision being made about treatment. Families were to be kept informed.

Everyone detained in hospital or treated within the community would require an individual care plan approved by a Tribunal or Court. When in care, patients retained the right to be involved in decisions about dangerous treatments such as psychosurgery or ECT. Here, the role of advocacy would be crucial. Patients could either nominate an Advocate to represent them at Tribunal or appear in person. Who these Advocates were, and how they were to be paid, remained a mystery.

Cost of Services

As you can imagine these measures would have cost a deal of money:
- training professionals in gate keeping roles
- training around the new Bill
- cost of community treatment centres
- cost of treatments in the community
- expenses connected with tribunals
- setting up costs

There was a great deal of ballyhoo about implementation whys and wherefores and how much funding would be poured into this project. What was never really explained was where the money was to come from.

Figure 16 How a Bill Becomes Law

House of Commons Readings
- Introduction of material to House of Commons
- 2nd reading in House of Commons - and debate
- Commons Committee stage; detailed scrutiny
- Commons Report Stage; further debate
- Commons 3rd reading - decision about the Bill

House of Lords Readings
- Introduction of material to House of Lords
- 1st reading
- House of Lords 2nd reading - and debate
- House of Lords Committee stage; scrutiny
- House of Lords Report Stage; further debate
- House of Lords 3rd reading; amendments
- Inter-House of Readings
- House of Commons amendments
- House of Lords amendments

Bill to / from House of Lords & Commons until agreed.

The Legislation Stage
- Royal Assent given
- Bill becomes an Act
- Act commences no less than 2 months later

Cue lights, cameras, action – get out your purse and look at tax returns! You can download the documents, arguments and counter-arguments from the websites of the Department of Health and any of the major mental health charity websites. Although this Bill has been discarded it is useful to know the history as there will be new legislation once current problems have been ironed out.

Updates on Mental Health Law

As I am no longer in the field, I do not feel in a position to comment on the following, as I have no access to professionals to check their views. The best I can do is provide web links [below] which give details and comment.

A Mental Capacity Act came into being in 2005. This website from the Mental health organization gives details:
http://www.mentalhealth.org.uk/help-information/mental-health-a-z/M/mental-capacity-act-2005/

This website gives a summary of the Mental Health Act 2007:
http://www.mentalhealthlaw.co.uk/Mental_Health_Act_2007

Here are articles by Community Care magazine, on the 1983 and 2007 Acts:
http://www.communitycare.co.uk/2008/11/11/mental-health-acts-1983-and-2007/

By way of respite, I offer a diversion. Readers who are unaware of how a Bill becomes law might care to read my synopsis (previous page) of the process. This applies to any kind of law. It appears repetitive, but this ensures nothing is missed and as many considerations as possible are given to new procedures to close potential loopholes (lacunae).

****

Key Learning
- Considerations - overriding considerations in mental health legislation are patient and public safety
- Patient Rights - it is useful to role play a scenario under which potential patient risk is balanced with human rights.

'People with mental disorders are some of the most neglected ..'
World Health Organization

8 THE WORLD HEALTH ORGANISATION

Content
The Mission of the World Health Organization (WHO)
Project Atlas

Do not believe your field only represents progress towards humane treatment of the mentally ill in the UK. There is much work to be done worldwide with some standards beggaring belief. All mental health workers need understand the field on a global basis not just the fractal of work in your area. It is good practice to do this.

When you complain about lack of budget or interest, searches on WHO or other mental health charity websites will put your complaints in context. As an example, I read of a mentally ill Indian woman locked in an outhouse by her family for her entire adult life. She could neither walk nor speak when she was rescued. Such inhumanity is by no means uncommon both in Eastern Europe and primitive cultures. In the Congo, one of the most deprived countries on earth population 2.5 million there is <u>one</u> psychiatrist. Read the story of Dr Alain Maxime Mouanga:
http://www.who.int/healthsystems/psychiatrist/en/index.html

Making a difference does not mean hurling money and resources at a project but looking what resources exist and their potential re-deployment. The armed forces, voluntary and local organizations are skilled in logistics and similar skills need to be deployed in the NHS. There is still dreadful waste, not only materials but infighting among professional factions and management systems which prevent co-operation between workers.

The World Health Organization (WHO) is a specialist section of the United Nations set up in 1948. Its headquarters are in Geneva and there are six offices across the globe. The aim of WHO is to enable complete physical, mental and social well-being.
ethical health policy-making, based on evidence
1. programmes of research
2. policies & programmes acceptable to member states
3. maintaining workable relationships in member states
4. conceiving, implementing & follow-through new health standards
5. gathering data on new technology and health care

Project Atlas

Contributing to the above report was Project Atlas. Readers will be interested to learn this massive project has been successfully completed. The value of having public statistics is enormous; pride for governments with minimal funding making best use of resources and shame where local governments have done little or nothing to help their mentally ill citizens.

Countries struggling to implement programmes in the face of financial limitations will be proud of their co-operation in this massive undertaking. The difficulties in obtaining statistics, bias factors (where government statistics alone are currently relied upon) and the problems of ensuring common language are gradually being resolved as the projects proceed.

****

WHO - The World Health Organisation website is an excellent place to get a feel for what is happening world wide in mental health. It is important to get a broader view than your own patch.

> 'Between 1940 and 1942, 70,723 mental patients were gassed, chosen..
> by 9 leading professors of psychiatry and 39 top physicians'
> Roy Porter, Madness, A Brief History

9 COMMUNITIES & MENTAL ILLNESS

Content
Effect of Living in Communities
Four Community Scenarios

Living in communities brings its own stresses which affect pre-existing conditions. I give myself as an example, as stress worsens the symptoms of autism, whereas peace reduces them. Those without mental conditions may not be aware of the extent to which well-functioning communities contribute to mental health.

Effect of Living in Communities
As well as ordinary life stress, attitudes to the mentally ill also affect their health. The fickle public tend to think of mental illness only when confronted with news reports of horrific murders, rape or the activity of paedophiles. This gives mentally ill people a negative image, affecting their social standing and status. Those with personality disorders are a tiny section of patients diagnosed with active mental illness, but the two are often un-distinguished in laymen's minds.

Mentally ill patients have heightened sensitivity and you might imagine patients loaded with embarrassment, shame and isolation, as well as their mental illness. Though some communities are welcoming, it takes few to dampen the atmosphere.

Rarely has illness of the mind been 'sexy' in the same way as cancer, child health or diet. I read an article in a national newspaper extolling the virtues of colonic irrigation, with an image of a Journalist publicly examining a basket of her doings. This was apparently acceptable to readers but mention mental illness and people will turn away. I offered the same newspaper an article for World Mental Health Day (10th October) but was ignored.

However, this head-in-the-sand trend is reversing as stars like Robbie Williams air their addictive peccadilloes in public. Where the famous lead, others follow. I see disclosure as healthy rather than unhealthy. The day a trendy star 'comes out' with schizophrenia, attitudes will change, among the young at least.

Effect of Living in Communities

Living in communities is stressful for most of us, with daily indignities, arguments, issues, errors and rebuttals. Imagine trying to cope with a physical or mental illness, or dual diagnosis, whilst dealing with the mores of ordinary daily life. I have witnessed, many times, people distraught at being forced to live in proximity of people who do not understand them, for whatever reason. I too have suffered in this way, for in my early life nothing was known of autism the greater number of individuals in the community. My brother suffered much the same way at school. Teasing or tormenting is what we now call bullying. It known to result in severe psychiatric injury which requires long-term, sometimes permanent treatment. Bullying exacerbates existing mental illness to a great degree, as can the social effects of exclusion (covered in the next chapter).

So why does such behaviour result in damage? It is because we are social creatures. Exclusion results in mental injury or even death. Rather cruel experiments were carried out on young chimps, deliberately separated from their mothers. Some actually died. This proved the devastating effects of shock to the nervous system, so this is scientific fact not fantasy.

In totalitarian states, isolation is a method of torture against so-called enemies of the state. Solitary confinement with enforced psychiatric medication leads to mental illness. If these prisoners are returned to their communities (if they are not murdered or commit suicide), they are known to suffer extreme anxiety, mistrust and other negative symptoms; symptoms which may last a lifetime.

Some are born into loving families, have friends and careers, but cannot cope with mental illness and succumb to despair or suicide because they cannot face more suffering. The recent death of Robin Williams shocked people all over the world. Here was outwardly a successful man, a great joker and clown, a fine actor, with many friends and loving family. Yet, he died alone in despair. A public face can hide a great deal, whether a fine movie star or a young person with a perceived great future.

Mental suffering equates to physical suffering. It is more insidious because it can neither be seen in the way of physical hurt. Such suffering rarely engenders sympathy, patience and kindness outside the small circle of family and friends but it is the reaction of the community that could make a difference. Whatever the issues, the fact remains that lack of public funding and interest on recognition and treatment of mental illness will prove costly, in terms of human suffering, and potentially fatal. Mental illness will not go away.

Figure 17   Perceptions of Individuals By Communities

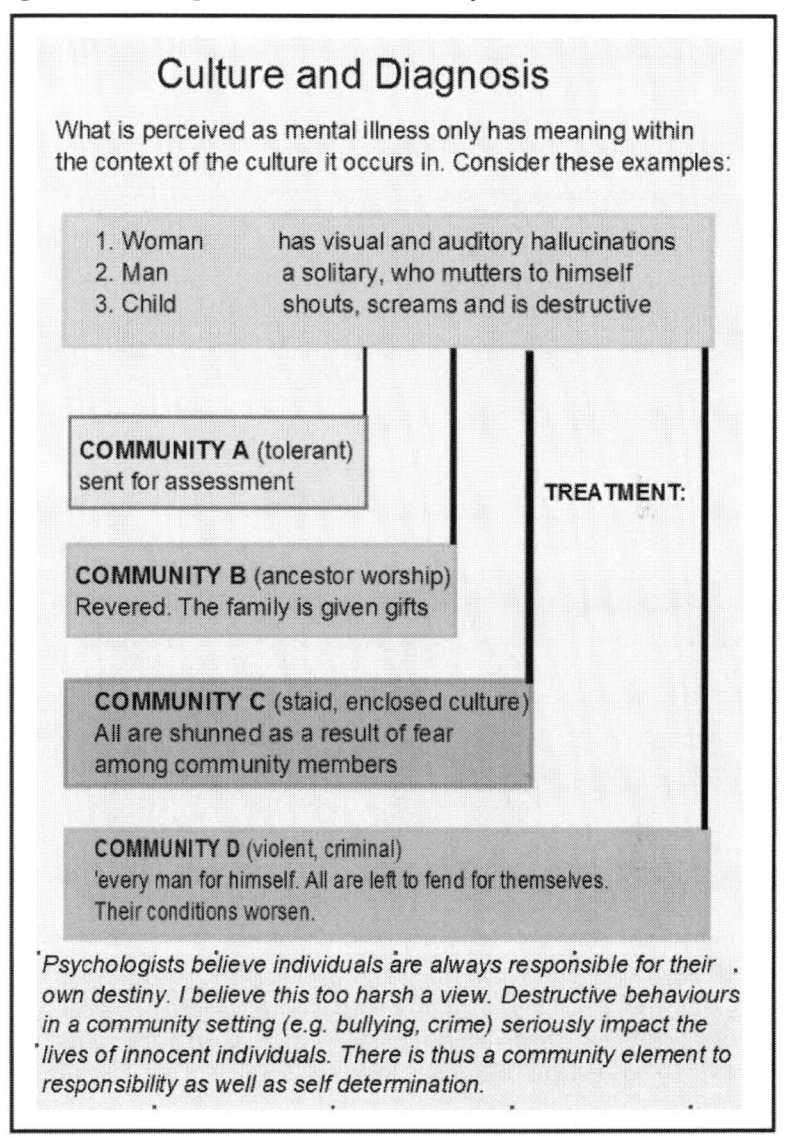

Culture and Diagnosis

What is perceived as mental illness only has meaning within the context of the culture it occurs in. Consider these examples:

1. Woman — has visual and auditory hallucinations
2. Man — a solitary, who mutters to himself
3. Child — shouts, screams and is destructive

COMMUNITY A (tolerant)
sent for assessment

TREATMENT:

COMMUNITY B (ancestor worship)
Revered. The family is given gifts

COMMUNITY C (staid, enclosed culture)
All are shunned as a result of fear among community members

COMMUNITY D (violent, criminal)
'every man for himself. All are left to fend for themselves. Their conditions worsen.

Psychologists believe individuals are always responsible for their own destiny. I believe this too harsh a view. Destructive behaviours in a community setting (e.g. bullying, crime) seriously impact the lives of innocent individuals. There is thus a community element to responsibility as well as self determination.

Four Community Scenarios

Consider these scenarios. Don't try to diagnose or judge these people; simply consider what would happen in the community where you live.
1. A woman experiences people whom no one else sees or hears.
2. A man mutters to himself, scratching his head until it bleeds.
3. A female child is reported to scream and shout every night

Let us consider four different styles of community.

In community A, all these people are seen as behaving strangely, but as members of this community are compassionate they are sent for observation, assessment and treatment.

In community B, where ancestors are revered, all three are revered as they are believed to be infused with the spirit of ancestors. Their families are given gifts and welcomed. They are not considered ill or insane and the community would be outraged if this was suggested.

In community C, people are afraid of these behaviours which they believe originate from bad spirits. The woman is hanged, the man exiled, the child is taken to an orphanage where a paedophile rapes her. In her teens she commits suicide.

In community D, there is violence and crime. The behaviours go unnoticed. The woman becomes psychotic and when a man comes towards her, she stabs and kills him. She is imprisoned for life. The man is followed by a taunting gang of youths. He commits suicide. The child is repeatedly hit by her parents. She runs away and is found wandering by a pimp (someone who lives off the earnings of prostitutes) who drugs her and forces her into prostitution. She is found unconscious in a squalid bedsit, dead, a dirty syringe and needle by her side.

Although the characters are fictitious, such circumstances exist. It it is the community which determines your ultimate fate.

Victoria Climbie Report

http://www.justiceinspectorates.gov.uk/hmic/media/victoria-climbie-inquiry-report-key-findings-20031009.pdf

I urge you to read the Victoria Climbie Enquiry which deals with the horrific torture and murder of a small child, because her relatives accused her of witchcraft. If you have no stomach for it, you should not be working in this field. Victoria was not mentally ill but a beautiful black child who lived in the wrong community. The Climbie Report must be compulsory reading for mental health workers. It is shocking these tragedies occur but only awareness will prevent them happening in future.

Figure 18 Victoria Climbie (RIP)
'The Victoria Climbie Inquiry: Report of an Inquiry' by Lord Laming January 2003.' *Victoria found dead in a bin liner, after being accused by relatives of practicing witchcraft. This child was first tortured then murdered.*

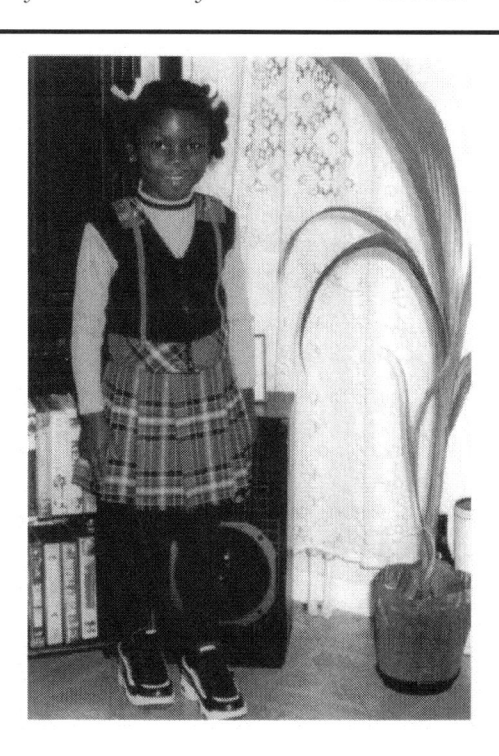

"I have suffered too much grief in setting down these heartrending memories. If I try to describe him, it is to make sure that I shall not forget him."

Jiro Hirabayashi from Yasunori Kawahara's
translation of *The Little Prince* by Antoine de Saint-Exupéry.

This sentiment applies also to Victoria Climbié.
This Report is dedicated to her memory.

https://www.gov.uk/government/uploads/system/uploads/attachment_data/file/273183/5730.pdf

Key Learning
- Community living & mental illness - Living in communities exacerbates existing mental illnesses or trigger conditions in formerly well people.
- Victoria Climbie & Bennett Reports - compulsory reading for mental health workers.
- Attitude/symptoms link - not only symptoms affect patients but attitudes to the mentally ill [see next chapter].

> "People who suffer from mental health problems remain one of the most excluded groups in society"
> Rosie Winterton, Health Minister

10 STIGMA & SOCIAL EXCLUSION

Content

David Bennett	Extermination of the Tutsi Tribe
Early Man & Identity	Poor Employer Tactics
Individuality as Threat	Barriers to Employability
The Seeds of Exclusion	Pressure at Work
Modern Ways with Anger	Fear of Misunderstanding
Stigma of Diagnosis	Erratic Course of Mental Illness
Stigma of Expressed Emotion	Barriers for Employers
Appearing Different	Mental Health Education
Stigma of Diagnosis	Living in Communities – summing up
Personal Effect of Exclusion	
Language of Exclusion	

A teacher of horticultural students with learning disabilities said on TV that though his students were ready for the community, the community was not yet ready for them. This applies equally to those with long term mental illness and for that matter autism. We are light years from the laid back attitudes of our cousins across the pond, because our communities remain rife with stigmatization. But in order to combat stigma, you need to understand what stigma is, how it manifests and where it originates. As a starting point: We need to go back in history and try to understand man in the context of his animal past, to discover connections between difference and stigma.

- humans exclude those who are different
- mental illness breeds social exclusion
- socially exclusion affects mental illness, potentially with long term scars

David Bennett

First a word about stigma among mental health workers. Another report which is required reading is the death of David Bennett, a Rastafarian with schizophrenia who died whilst under restraint by five nurses, after attacking another patient. Though David was under a delusion he was being attacked by racists, the inquiry concluded '..*that institutional racism has been present in the mental health services, both NHS and private, for many years*' (refer website: http://www.irr.org.uk/pdf/bennett_inquiry.pdf

Racism among staff is abhorrent and deserves a mention in this section. The nurses were stressed as a colleague had been seriously injured by

David, nevertheless it was concluded there was too much restraint, too many nurses restraining - and a strong sense of people acting out shadow emotions.

So stigmatization here comes from an unexpected quarter. Nurses are not immune from negative traits, though expected to perform as if they are perfect beings. This report and the tragic ending is surely a grave lesson, that stigmatization DOES affect people, that wounds go deep and that years of torment often have violet conclusions. David suffered years of racial torment that went so deep it was ingrained in his psyche, bursting out during his psychosis in a way that brought catastrophe to himself and his family and shock waves among the staff and their colleagues. It is not only the act itself but the repercussions - and that is a valuable lesson to remember.

But where did such aggressive hatred of others originate? What was the purpose? It stems from our animal nature, our animal past that has not developed down the generations. But why?

Early Man and Identity

Thousands of years ago, man learned that group co-operation lead to more successful hunting and better survival. And so they began to live in groups. Over time, man discovered how to cultivate crops and corral animals to provide readily available food. Instead of a nomadic life, with most of the day spent hunting, at last there was time for each man to specialize, to hone skills in one particular niche rather than learning all the survival skills. This was the beginning of personal identity. Archaeologists have discovered fine artwork, jewelry and factories where small groups of men made spear throwers, axes and arrowheads, trading this for skins, jewelry and other commodities. This could not have happened if each was a lone hunter, concerned only with his own survival.

These tribes lived in a fragile, hostile world. Burials prove that ritual became as important as hunting. Now, some men became religious leaders, shamans, or organizers of labour. These administrators oversaw the building of great monuments like Avebury or Stonehenge. Life became complex even as it became safer, for men now lived in close proximity. Loss of individual survival skills would have meant that it would be virtually impossible for each man to survive on his own. But there was another problem.

We know animals in overcrowded conditions fight and some practice cannibalism. The mainly vegetarian ape family was no different. We do not know when these tribes developed morality, apart from careful burials which included grave goods and imply mourning. Neither do we know if some ritual sacrifices were in fact murders. Here were the beginnings of stigma. Individuality brings challenges, as young apes challenge silverbacks.

Figure 19 David Bennett, RIP

'Independent Inquiry into the death of David Bennett', Dec 2003
http://www.irr.org.uk/pdf/bennett_inquiry.pdf

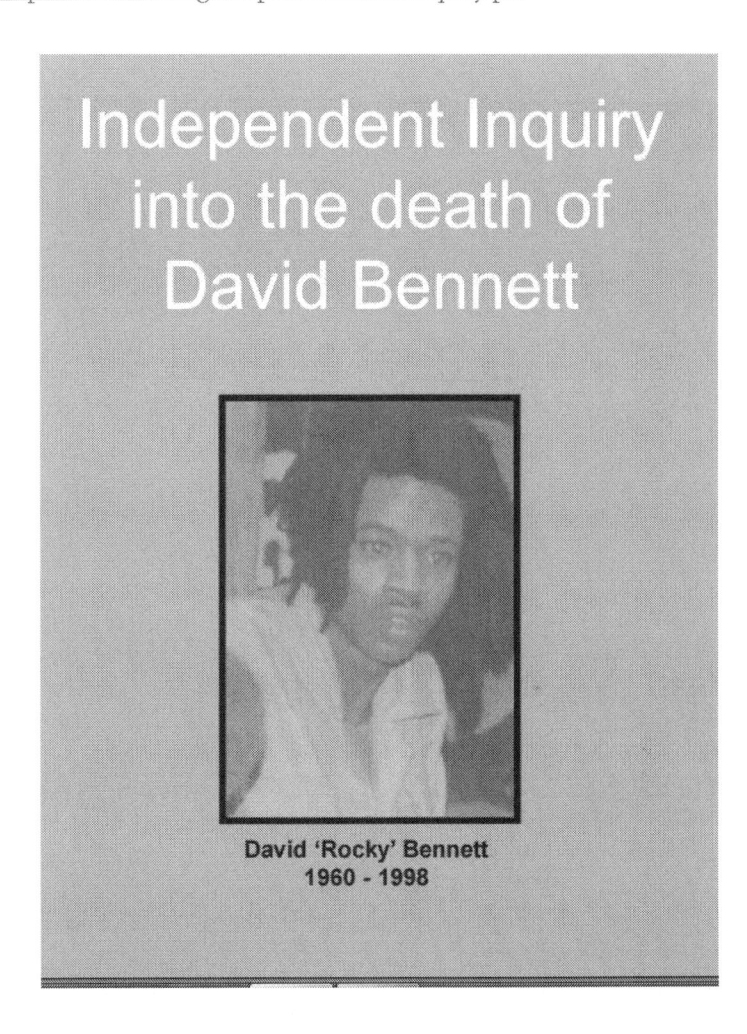

Independent Inquiry into the death of David Bennett

David 'Rocky' Bennett
1960 - 1998

'We have concentrated in this report on how to prevent injury to the patient because, in the case of David Bennett, he died while under restraint.'

At the dawn of civilization, individuals began a journey towards settled communities, yet there were not immune to the same shadows that haunt communities today; stigma, roles and skills that lead to envy, greed or desire for dominance.

Individuality as Threat

Individuality breeds vulnerability. What if the shaman leaves, dies or joins another tribe? If tribe members do not know how to make magic or good tools they are in danger, vulnerable to attack from wild animals as well as other tribes. If an individual loses his range of skills through lack of practice, he is likely to die if rejected by the group. There must have been inter-group rivalries, a trait shared with pack animals like wolves or jackals. Natural rivalries would influence potential rejection. In other words, social differences were beginning to emerge might contain seeds of the group's destruction, real or perceived threats from within or outside the group:

- leadership threat (inside threat)
- potential magicians taking over (perceived inside threat)
- distant rival tribal group (outside threat)
- group living close by (perceived outside threat)

Early man was as intelligent as homo sapiens but this intellect was limited to the environment of the time. Nature was to primitive man a raw and dangerous force, highly unpredictable. Perhaps we take for granted the scientific principles which allow us relative control over the environment, or at least the possibility of early warning and sophisticated search and rescue equipment. The overriding sense of primitive man was fear of the unknown – volcanoes erupting, storms, tsunamis, crop failure, the death of herd animals, rivers drying up or sudden changes in climate. Knowledge is power and though natural events cannot be manipulated we know how to tame and survive them, in the main.

The Seeds of Exclusion

Early tribal leaders were powerful magicians who were believed to communicate and intercede with nature gods. Such men directed the course of the tribe's life. If they disliked or feared someone and could not be appeased, the tribe member risked being murdered or cast out. (This begins to sound like toxic work places with narcissist managers..)

Humans of course have positive and negative characteristics. These developed long before history bred morality. Envy, spite, fear, greed, suspicion, aggression, drive to destroy, fear of the unknown are raw instincts which account for discontent and wars. Powerful feelings are easily projected on individuals perceived as somehow different, objects of fear or targets of envy. In modern times, negative emotions are connected with possessions, talent and wealth than the nice raw carcass of a kill. Older men fear being displaced; younger members want power or fear the power of stronger men.

Personal confidence (strength) can appear challenging in a group that is vulnerable, more so than in groups where individuals have a sense of worth and environmental security. In weaker or fearful groups lacking leadership, those perceived as stronger might become targets for exclusion or assassination because of fear. So to sum up:

- confident groups and individuals are less likely to reject
- vulnerable groups and insecure individuals more so
- fear can express itself as anger, aggression and rejection
- difference in organizations can lead to targeting

These are the seeds of rivalries whether religious, sporting, ethnicity, looks, disability or racial.

Modern Ways of Expressing Anger

Modern man has the opportunity to release the anger or envy of rivalry in more positive outlets:

- sporting or team activity
- artistic achievement and competition
- healthy ethnic or cultural allegiances
- cross cultural understanding
- humour

Sadly, man is not always as rational as he is capable of becoming. He is also more subtle in his negative behaviours. Rather than pick a fight, he might incite others or find a scapegoat, as politicians or managers often do.

Moral panics are a modern phenomena, when a group 'blames' an individual or group for their ills. For examples, Jews were blamed by German Nazis for poverty in Germany in the 1930's. At one time, gypsies were vilified in the press, so too single mothers and of course that perennial target, mentally ill people.

Why Stigmatization

It is easy to understand why patients who look odd or act strangely to become targets. These are some myths about mental illness;

- a belief those with mental illness might be murderous
- that mental illness is somehow infectious - like a virus
- lack of knowledge leads to false conjectures
- fear of 'exposure by association'

The real problem is not the illness but how it is perceived. Symptoms of mental illness cannot be seen except through behaviour and/or emotion. The unseen is always the most powerfully stigmatized and there are few means of redressing such fears.

Appearing Different

Some patients with chronic (long term) mental illness, talk to themselves, dress strangely, exhibit tics (uncontrollable muscle spasms), shout at no one in particular (hearing voices). This was particularly so when medications were not as effective as they are today. Tics were caused by chemicals in early medication, for example tongue and lip smacking (tardive dyskinesia), grimacing or shaking.

Strange or old fashioned clothing was a hallmark for patients who had been in hospital for decades wearing communal clothing. Those with chronic illness were too ill to be aware of appearance. Young patients may love fashion and be aware of trends, but have no cash to indulge in clothing. These factors faced pioneering patients thrust out of their secure Asylum homes and into the community in the 1990's.

The Stigma of Diagnosis

A physical symptom is relatively easily diagnosed. A General Practitioner (GP) has physical clues to aid diagnosis; lumps, swellings, bruising, spots, broken bones. Mental illness diagnoses are more difficult to make and even then patients and relatives will be reluctant to accept diagnosis. Behaviour, emotions and feelings are hard to quantify and measure unless the patient is obviously psychotic, depressed or manic.

Stigma of Highly Expressed Public Emotions

Patients who are psychotic have no insight into their behaviour and can easily become angry or upset. Even neurotic patients find it difficult to 'see' changes that brought them to a GP or Psychiatrist, because insight disappears during heightened emotion. Think of times you were distressed and did not realize, until someone pointed it out, how angry or tearful or detached you had become.

Whilst highly expressed emotion is accepted in the case of pregnancy, birth, bereavement or divorce, prolonged emotion in public places is still taboo. The dys-inhibitions of mental illness are particularly visible and mark out vulnerable patients for attack or ridicule.

Personal Effect of Exclusion

Community life is good for those find it easy to join in. Patients with severe mental illness who have been hospitalized long term do not have social skills; either they have never learned them, forgotten how or have received dysfunctional parenting. Even those who live in the community and have their symptoms controlled by medications will find it difficult to socialize and so become known to other people around them. Sadly, the community does not always live up to its name or ideals. Very few people will ask others to join in. Those with family are generally so wrapt up and busy that they find little time to welcome others. This means social isolation for many, including those without mental illness.

Social isolation is, as we have seen, very damaging to physical health as well as the mental state. Think of those experimental monkeys deprived of their mothers, most of whom died. And socially isolated people are too easily targeted, as I have explained.

The language of Exclusion

The language we use when referring to those diagnosed with mental illness affects very strongly how they are perceived. Some historic language causes offence, though at the time the words did not have the same pejorative meanings. These terms were used to describe anyone who showed bizarre behaviour before mental illness was understood:

- mad
- lunatic
- insane

Some terms have been used in jocular fashion, such as young people calling mates psycho or crazy. Perhaps it is pertinent to ask such persons if they would like being called fat, stupid or ignorant. Historically, name calling is used by unscrupulous people, from gangs to totalitarian states, as the first stage in belittling or isolating individuals, groups or nations, prior to wiping them out. One only has to think of examples from recent history:

Extermination of Tutsi Tribe

The Hutu and Tutsi tribes were traditional enemies of long standing. Hutu's at one time had been an underclass and cultivated a desire for revenge. In 1994, there was a massacre of the Tutsis in which half a million people were murdered using machetes. This massacre had been well organised. Millions of refugees were fearful of returning to their country of birth. The emotional scars are there to this day, though much work has been and is being done to redress the traumas.

Jews, Gypsies, Disabled and Mentally Ill

Lead by Hitler, German Nazis subjected Jews, Gypsies, disabled and mentally ill people to pograms; they were murdered in their millions through starvation, the gas chamber and assassination by the SS.

Ordinary German working people had been convinced that these were racially impure people who had degenerated the pure Aryan gene pool.

These outcast people were blamed for Germany's low status.

Low Self Esteem

Having read so far you may realize how people with mental illness often undervalue themselves. To undervalue yourself is to reduce your human potential. I have seen this in many people I met during my career; 'if only I didn't have this illness..' Having the illness is bad fortune but not having the opportunity to gain happiness then being excluded is tragedy.

Poor Employer Tactics

A survey carried out in 2001 by Focus found seventy five percent of people with mental illness considered they were on low income and led a frills free, isolated existence. A large proportion of those with long standing mental illness are unable to do, or excluded from, jobs which reflect their academic ability, creativity or other skills.

People with mental illness might come to the career market late in life if at all. If they have a CV with long periods of unemployment (often mistaken by employers for periods in prison) they fall into the temporary work trap. Many agencies offer work which commands high fees from corporate clients but pays below the market rate for the job. They call this cheap labour 'flexible work' or 'contracting' or 'getting into the labour market'.

There are few employment laws in temporary work yet agencies earn billions of pounds per year through this most profitable human traffic. Agencies, as I know from experience, are clever at hiding facts from researchers. They claim workers 'insist' or 'love' working on temporary contracts or 'feel freer' to work on zero hour contracts. Do people really love irregular income, irregular work and low pay? Once workers are trapped in this system, by dint of months or years on 'temporary' contracts, it is very difficult for them to obtain permanent work. And these are the most vulnerable of the workforce.

Over time, many trad firms are also offering zero hours contracts, where workers are expected to take no other job but wait around until their 'contracted' employer calls them in. Another abuse of labour are the growing number of 'voluntary' jobs or 'internships'. They offer 'experience' or expenses in return for free labour. This takes a number of jobs, particularly in the charity sector, out of the paid labour market. Once this got a strong-hold in the charity sector (perhaps where you might least expect it), it ran rampant. Another clever trick was persuading middle class students to pay for their own travel and accommodation, and calling their efforts 'fund raising' and 'an experience.' Mental health charities are getting wise to this and starting to demand better conditions for service users.

MENTAL ILLNESS & THE COMMUNITY vol 1

Figure 20 Contributory Factors to Mental Illness

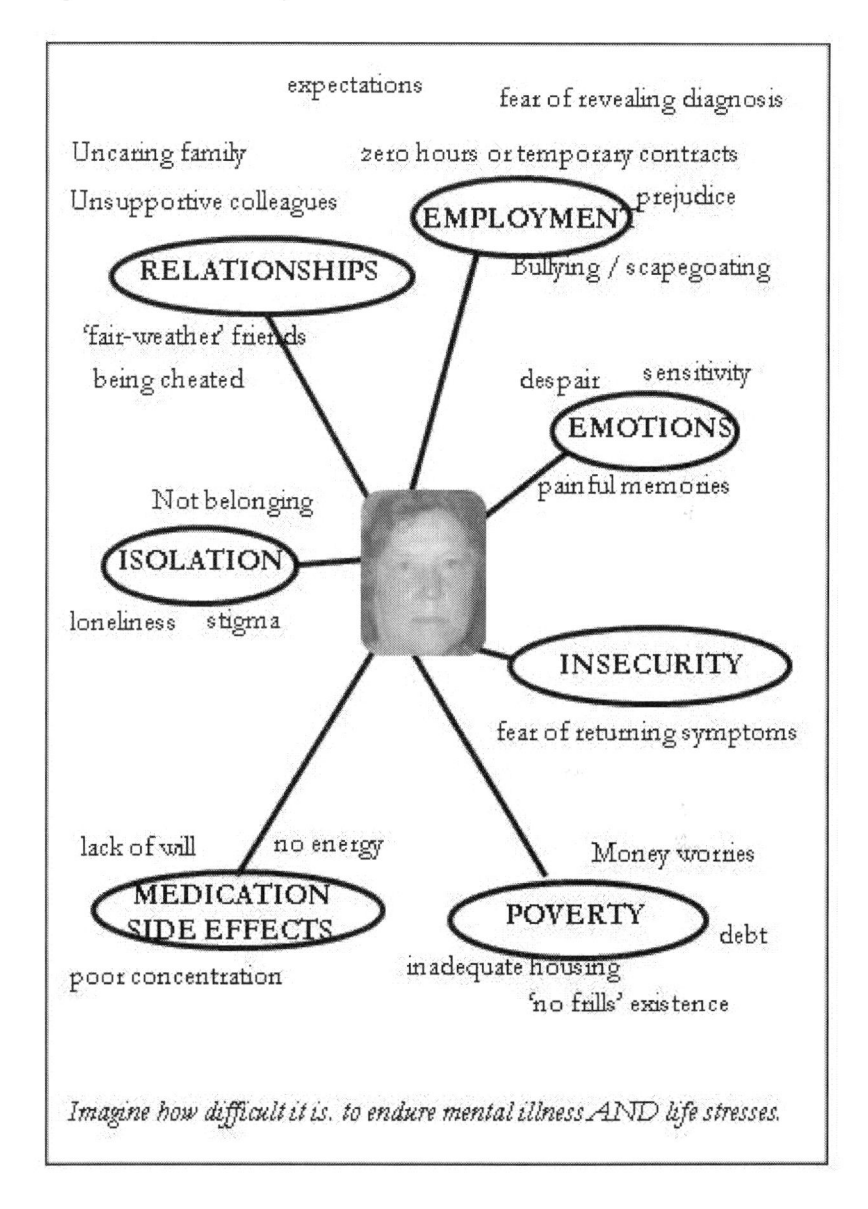

expectations
fear of revealing diagnosis
Uncaring family
zero hours or temporary contracts
Unsupportive colleagues
EMPLOYMENT
prejudice
RELATIONSHIPS
Bullying / scapegoating
'fair-weather' friends
being cheated
despair   sensitivity
EMOTIONS
painful memories
Not belonging
ISOLATION
loneliness   stigma
INSECURITY
fear of returning symptoms
lack of will   no energy
Money worries
MEDICATION SIDE EFFECTS
POVERTY
debt
poor concentration
inadequate housing
'no frills' existence

Imagine how difficult it is. to endure mental illness AND life stresses.

Huxley commented with humour that funding agencies of his day existed to prevent those who need the money most from getting it. The situation has not changed. It is a fact that no one on benefits can afford to pay thousands of pounds to train in a profession and are thus trapped in underpaid and highly stressful warehousing or shop work. I wonder if it has changed much since George Orwell wrote Down and Out in London and Paris or The Road to Wigan Pier. This is intelligence left to rot in grubby towns and dingy bedsits and in the 21st century this is scandalous.

Barriers to Employability

There are barriers from the job seeker's point of view and there are barriers from the employer's point of view. If someone does not have professional qualifications they are likely to stay in the poverty trap unless artistically successful or turn to crime as a career. People with mental illness are competing against others who are not so disadvantaged. Perhaps, like my brother with a Mensa level IQ, they might be offered a job as a cleaner on a Government sponsored scheme. Many people, even professionals, tend to forget there is an intellectual ability trapped inside symptoms which label a man or a woman 'depressive' or 'schizo' or 'autistic'.

Pressure at Work

There will be times when someone with active mental illness needs time off, but a neuro typical will need time off too. Structures need to be in place to ensure there is support through Occupational Health. One idea emerging is mentoring or buddying.

Anyone who has been out of work on long term sick leave will experience much the same anxieties as someone with mental illness. In most companies there is more work than paid man-hours as a result of cost-cutting which results in considerable stress for staff. This can pile on the stress for someone with existing mental health problems.

Fear of Misunderstanding

The existing workforce is generally as ignorant of mental illness as the rest of the population which is surprising given 1:4 people will develop mental illness during their lifetime. This could be resolved by providing mental health education at an early stage, a task the Government has started to undertake on a large scale where it counts, at Primary School level.

Bullying is common in the workplace (25% to 50%). People with mental illness are obvious targets with emotional insecurities, strange behaviours and lack of street wisdom. No one wants to go out to work and find they are in a worse state of mental health than before they went.

Erratic Course of Mental Illness

Staff can consult DSMV (diagnostics and statistics manual), perhaps thanks to brain scanning they might be able to point with accuracy to where brain chemistry is causing a problem. They might, thanks to the unravelling of the human genome (DNA sequence) be able to give you the number of the sequence or the name of the hormone causing the problem. What they cannot yet do is say when you are likely to experience an episode of mental illness or how you will experience it (in emotional or behavioural terms).

The erratic course of mental illness, and inability to predict when episodes might occur, make employment more hazardous and risky both to employers and potential employees (outside social enterprises). However, if you look at the figures for sickness and stress the same could be said for a large chunk of the population.

Barriers for Employers

Barriers exist on the other side too; that of potential employers. There is the question of unknown quantity. Employers have to consider existing staff and how they might react to colleagues who are different. It can be, as my friend commented, like putting a giraffe in a herd of elephants. I experienced this myself many times over the years, which is why I feel qualified to write about these issues.

Within the creative industry there tends to be more tolerance otherwise you would not have been able to enjoy talents of DJ Kenny Everett or actor Jeremy Brett (Granada's Sherlock Holmes for over a decade) both of whom had well publicized mental illness.

These are by no means all the reasons why mentally ill patients are social excluded whether they have long term episodic illness or a one-off attack. But what are we doing about this?

Mental Health Education

Mental health education initiatives are being started where they should have been years ago; in primary schools, in communities, in surgeries.

Mental health for everyone is a Government priority with recent figures showing mental illness and stress to be the number one reason for sickness absence in this country - a sobering thought. Mental health charities are as always doing great work in this area, under-funded, under staffed and under resourced as they remain.

The major problem is that mental health education initiatives are not sexy news and never will be. However, if you look at some Channel 4 documentaries, the ones on caring, there is good work being done through the creative media.

Living in Communities – Summing Up

Living in a community is not easy. Reading an individual's meaning is difficult. Imagine the number of times you made assumptions about someone, only for that view to be blown away as you got to know the person behind the diagnosis. Multiply this by thousands, all with pathology, personal agendas and issues. When you add mental illness into this murky soup the potential for damage is colossal, to the patient, family and friends and community at large. This represents a huge loss of talent, skill and manpower, to say nothing of individual happiness.

****

Key Learning

- Early Man & Social Exclusion - social exclusion began as soon as individuality emerged in early man.
- mentally ill patients are often at a disadvantage in the job market, for many reasons, and this adds to their distress
- Education reduces exclusion - much exclusion is the result of lack of knowledge or information.
- Mental health education is a vital tool to prevent exclusion
- there are many barriers to employment, including lack of funding for proper training
- many of the lower skilled among the workforce are exploited by temporary agencies and charities offering only voluntary work
- all this represents a huge loss to the community at large

Figure 21 Origin of Scapegoats

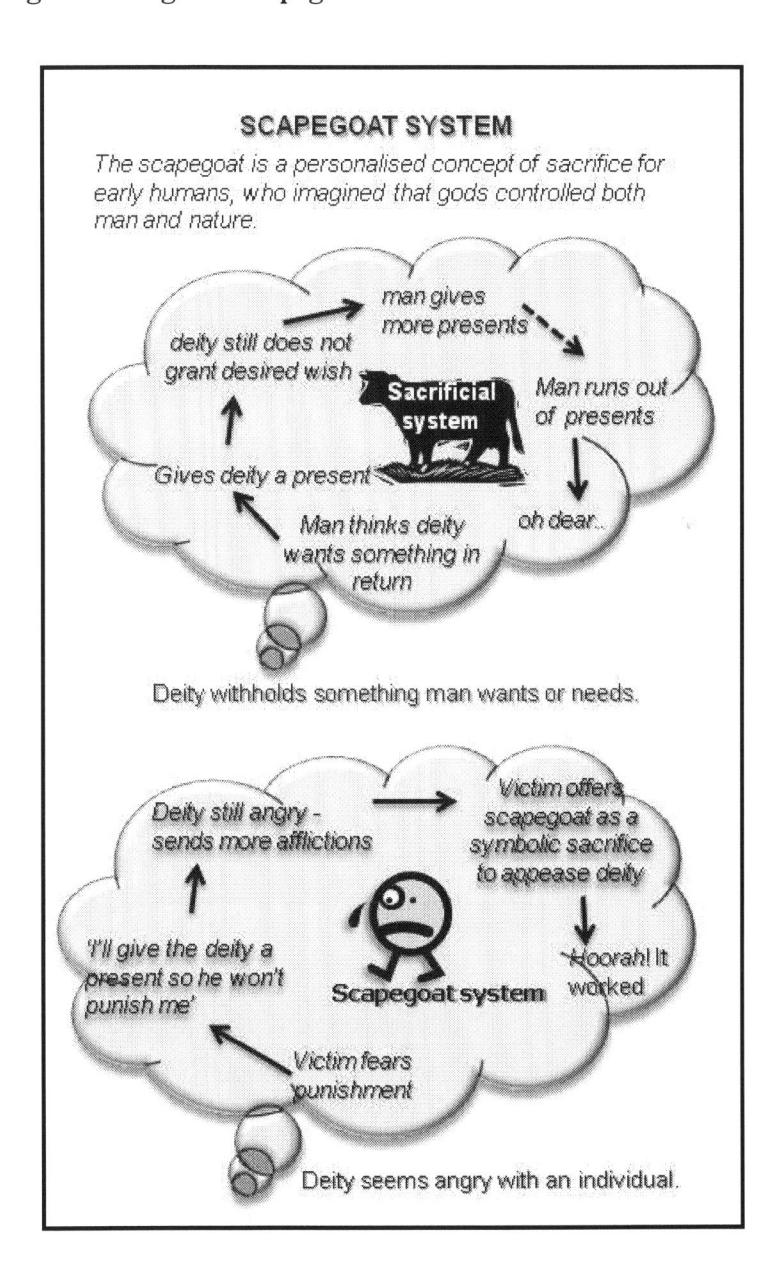

> "I attribute the little I know to my not having been ashamed to ask for information [and] conversing with **all** descriptions of men.."
>
> John Locke

11 REDUCING SOCIAL EXCLUSION

Content
Who is Responsible for Social Exclusion
Changing Symbolic Language
What Can Improve Social Inclusion?
Paid and Interesting Work
Mental Health Clubs
Mental Health Workers and Inclusion

Who is Responsible for Social Exclusion
The answer to this question is; all of us. We all have prejudices whether or not we admit it. Influence comes from many sources:

- strong charismatic personalities (Hitler, Gandhi, Buddha)
- schools (copied attitudes)
- family attitudes (what is learned in the early years)
- communities (peer pressure is very strong)
- faith organisations
- work colleagues
- media - powerful attitude formers
- movies and fiction
- books and magazines
- the media
- the Internet
- groups, clubs, organizations

Man is a social animal but at times is suspicious and easily influenced. As the only animals with consciousness (awareness), so far as we are aware, man is equipped to learn and change. Learning and changing is where social exclusion will change. So, let's change the word exclusion for inclusion be positive and see what we can **all** do to improve matters.

Changing Symbolic Language
The language of stigma is negative and breeds contempt, mistrust and ridicule. By way of example, let us consider Jo[e] Smith, who lives in a small town. Jo[e] is a creative person but has developed schizophrenia in his [her] late teens. Jo[e] has friends both inside and outside the mental health

community. Imagine you are Jo[e] – look at the table on the next page, and consider how you would like to be addressed.

Figure 22   The Language of Stigma

Negative:	Positive:
He's a schizo	Jo[e] has schizophrenia
Jo[e]s gone psycho	Jo[e]'s ill at the moment
He's a misery guts	Jo[e]'s depressed
That oddball Jo[e]	Jo[e]'s just a bit different
I hate being with him	Jo[e] is my colleague

Words matter. Don't let anyone convince you otherwise. People with mental illness are <u>people</u> first, not a diagnosis. They are neighbours, friends, relatives, confidantes, colleagues; part of the community you live in.

What Can Improve Social Inclusion?

Everyone can do something, absolutely everyone. I am not the only person with ideas, nor are mental health charities or professionals. Social inclusion is not about someone else doing something, it is YOU doing something, even changing a hard-wired attitude. I gave a list of ideas in my last book Understanding Mental Illness so will not repeat them. As mental health workers you need to work it out yourselves.

Paid and Interesting Work

For work to be meaningful, it has to fulfill three functions:

- provide a genuine product or service
- a sense of fulfillment and achievement
- a sense of belonging (identity)

Totalitarian states provide work for all, by making their unemployed dig ditches and fill them in. This is not genuine employment. Neither is voluntary work on a permanent basis, unless the volunteer has sufficient income to support themselves in a reasonable lifestyle and not a frills-free existence. Everyone has the right to feel respected, by society at large and have their skills and experience recognized.

I know huge numbers of people who work in dull, underpaid jobs which are often dangerous, lack career structure or are unfulfilling. Most people have choices. Those with major mental illness have not, for they face huge barriers from colleagues and employers alike.

Mental Health Clubs

I talked in my last book about the positive and negative faces of mental health clubs; how they could provide support but at the same time can turn into ghettos which encourage institutionalization and prevent people trying to join in community activity. Very severely ill mental health patients find them useful in breaking the monotony of the day, but with the advent of effective medication, I believe this will become less the case, particularly if social conditions improve.

Mental Health Workers and Inclusion

Mental Health Workers prime task is to integrate and educate, however that is achieved. There are many ways to do this. Inclusion will only come slowly and I mean changes in the attitudes of staff too. Sadly there will probably be more deaths and sadness before that happens.

I can only repeat Mother Teresa's fine expression; all change happens one person at a time.

Key Learning

- Education - mental health education from an early age is a vital key to social inclusion and prevention of stigmatisation.
- Responsibility - we all share responsibility for social inclusion.

> 'I know not with what weapons World War III will be fought, but World War IV will be fought with sticks and stones'
> Albert Einstein

12 Epilogue

I hope you have found this book useful and now have a little more knowledge at your fingertips to do further research. Volume 2 of this series covers diagnosis, treatments and case histories; how a patient is brought for treatment, how therapists carry out their work and what happens next.

This is an ever changing field so it is necessary to constantly revise and update your knowledge to take account of new trends. I hope you have realized how closely treatment is tied up with public opinion about the supposed causes of mental illness and this too has a bearing on how patients are treated.

At the best of times, communities can be volatile places which are stressful to live in, but modern man is blessed and cursed by this factor.

Rachel's Challenge

I can't think of a better way of ending than direct you to a website I came across whilst researching social exclusion. You might the massacre at Columbine High School. The first student to be murdered was 17 year old Rachel. Rachel had written a remarkable essay several years before she died which contained the following advice to readers:

- ♥ Eliminate prejudice by looking for the best in others
- ♥ Dare to dream. Write down goals, and keep a journal
- ♥ Choose positive influences. Input determines output
- ♥ Do acts of kindness
- ♥ Start a chain reaction

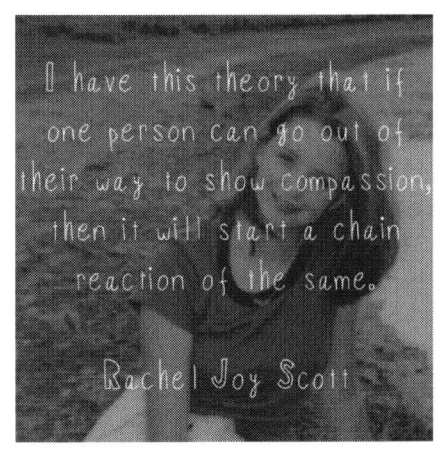

> I have this theory that if one person can go out of their way to show compassion, then it will start a chain reaction of the same.
>
> Rachel Joy Scott

There can be no finer challenge to Mental Health Workers than to follow Rachel's legacy. http://rachelschallenge.org/

Appendix 1 Potential for a new NHS model in the UK?

DR SUSAN PARENTI NEW MODEL HEALTH CARE SYSTEM FOR THE US
http://www.patchadams.org/re-designing-us-health-care-system/

"The first position is the status quo: the health care system as developed by entrenched health system industries (hospital, insurance, pharmaceutical, information technologies—with government primarily acting as their watchdog). The medical profession of doctor—its history of professional sovereignty—now no longer provides the bottom line in health care. The bottom line belongs to a different bottom: Big Business. We add a third position—whole system design—our frontline, can-do position: **Do it local, do it now, do it small, link with all.**

Given that there's a call for fundamental change in the US health care system, we respond by saying---that means, design something that DOESN'T act like a corporation.

PERTURBATION
Perturbation is the action of desperate and thoughtful people.
Perturbations are ideas/actions that put the system on the spot with the aim of destabilizing it, of making it trip on itself. When thinking of perturbations, we aim at the system's moving itself in a new direction under its own weight and inertia, as it attempts to compensate for our putting it on the spot. This is different from reforming or improving a system, where we aim at ourselves moving the system.

We turn to perturbation when we humbly admit that folks, we're in a David-and-Goliath position here as regards to change of health care system, in that:
1. the system we want to change is in the control of people/institutions who have power over us;
2. the system as is—unchanged—benefits them enormously;
3. these people/institutions have no intention of allowing change of that system, no matter how reasonable and ethical the arguments for change, no matter how compelling the evidence of human suffering and human waste, no matter how many compromises activists are willing to make towards these people/institutions.

In terms of perturbation, we do have a chance: the health care system in the US is so big, so complicated, so bureaucratic, with parts unable to connect to other parts, so insensitive to the mood of its environment, so unable to see its consequences—that falling by means of its own weight is a possibility.

Do we have a choice about anything in health care systems? Yes. Where we have a choice, there we can design.

1.   Health care interactions inherit a culture of hierarchy, rank abuse, posing. This is something a group of people, in shaping their health care facility along the lines they want, can support, oppose, change, alter. — this is something that can be designed

2.   In our consumerist culture, health/sickness is identified as being an individual property—a person sees her health as her own individual state, she battles against her disease, alone. (This, in the face of many studies that show a person has better health outcomes if she feels her wellbeing integrated within that of a larger group.) A group of healers/designers can come up with a language—frames and metaphors—that oppose this isolationist consumerist tendency, and situate the health of the individual with the health of a group. —this is something that can be designed

3.   Health of the staff as important as the health of the patient —this is something that can be designed

4.   **Participating in health as a people's popular movement** Commercial culture names a patient as consumer and a doctor/nurse as provider. Given this framing, health care interactions are experienced as a form of shopping, for both patients and healers. Beyond stopping at the counter to get a pill, patients in the United States do not participate in health, health care, or health care systems. Designers can oppose this state of affairs and make elements in their facility (**by means of language, imagery, structure**) that enable popular participation in all aspects/levels of health, health care, and health care system. —this is something that can be designed

5.   **Nesting** Currently health care has been nested in bureaucratic and financial institutions. This can be counter-acted: healing interactions need to be protected by nesting them in larger *beneficial* social groups. —this is something that can be designed

6.   **Solidarity** We need to rescue the concept/feeling/action of solidarity from North America's garbage heap. In the current culture, each person feels "you're on your own", "everyone for himself". Thus under-staffing of nurses is experienced as the nurses' problem, not the problem of the doctor, medical student, patient, family, technician. This reveals a lack of solidarity between people whose interests are fundamentally in common. This reveals that the lines of solidarity need

to be refreshed and redrawn. There need to be discussions about whose interests are being represented. Does the design move in the direction toward creating constructs in which solidarity between the greatest number of different people/groups is supported? —this is something that can be designed

7. **Decision-making** Who makes decisions? Is decision-making about health care system dilemmas communicated to/from the people? Does the health care system *listen*, in addition to *talk*? —this is something that can be designed

8. **Communication** How is information communicated and disseminated? Where is it? —to be designed

9. **Motivation of actors** Who stands to benefit? In whose interests are decisions made? Are the motivations of the others clear to each? Differences of power? —to be designed

10. Do people seek out health care, or does health care come to them? Is the health care system visible only when a sick person looks for it, or does a person have the sense she is nested in care? —to be designed

11. **Cure or care?** In the health care facility, is there a behavior which values cure over a commitment to care? —to be designed

12. **Spaces** Does the space (rooms, hallways, waiting rooms) support the values we want? —to be designed

13. **Presentation of self in everyday life** The way healers, staff, and patients act in everyday life is a choice and can be a tremendously valuable input to desirable health care interactions. There is no neutral interaction. —to be designed

The health care crisis is, amongst other things, a crisis of bankrupt ideas. People recognize that things need to change; they do not recognize that something has to be *made up*.

THE ANSWERS

Systems are circular; something which seems to be a cause turns out to be an effect of something else, and so on. Where to start?

If a system of **one payer, single tier, universal access** is created, then hopefully that will lead to a significant change in many other aspects of the culture of care in the system.

Designs where the **health care relation *shapes* the system, and where the system *protects* the relation**. If a group of health care providers at a clinic are involved in designing their practice, our hope is that a change in the culture of care will open the way to a change in the funding of it, or at least make people more susceptible to that change.

We say—local initiatives for the good of the public renew the sense of confidence in a group of people governing. **Campaign universally, design locally.**

Our strategy is this—rather than priding ourselves in working with organized business, we want to oppose and **expose the undesirability of market-controlled health care** and to **popularize a hands-off-health care**, corporations!! sentiment in Americans and in business-people themselves.

The abundance of bureaucracy in the medical system—the paperwork, the overseeing of diagnostic decisions by insurance companies, etc.—is not an error in the system. It is the *intended consequence* of the current system. **The system is being maintained at the expense of the well being of its members.**

Talking Points
1. We question at every opportunity the appropriateness of market capitalism to control (nest) the delivery of health care. We discuss the limits of free markets and the need for non-market regulation of experiential goods (a term in economics for services whose outcome is uncertain). We point out that in the case of a relationship dominated good such as health care, cutting costs in overhead results in cutting care itself.
2. We debate the assumption that health care is (needs must be) expensive. The expense of health care is not a property of health care in itself; the expense is an engineered condition, a consequence of the present design. We debunk the framing that health care will always be costly by making reference to counter-examples.
We invite media and wireless activists to demonstrate how the use of technology in health care can be free.

Every time the question, "Who will pay for this expensive system" is asked, we balance this with our question, "Who has been profiting such that this system is expensive?"

Health care, by its nature, is inexpensive—it's primarily a relationship along with some tools. We keep that image in mind so that we avoid playing into the assumptions of the market. The "high cost of care", the "complexity of the system" are frames that fuel the symbolic capital of the current system.
3. We caution that when big business says "we're committed to cutting

costs in health care" this DOES NOT mean "we're committed to making health care inexpensive". It doesn't mean that. Within market capitalism cutting costs means lowering overhead (workers' wages, resources) to keep profit at margins attractive to investment capital. It *does not* refer to lowering the cost of health care so that it's easily available to us who need it. Market forces always say they want to cut costs; the question of reducing their profit margins is never brought up.

4. We rename the health care system the 'disease management system'. When a person gets into the medical system, that person is getting disease management not health care. Disease management is a far smaller domain than the domain of health care. Health care is a huge domain of interactions, happening primarily outside the medical system, available to all, only not organized. John Glick, MD says, "Every moment is a health care moment". When does health care start? — when you decide to take a walk early in the morning? When you feel like you're getting a cold and a friend gives you Echinacea drops in a cup of tea?

What is health care at its indispensible minimum? Against the noise tunnel of the expensive and complicated disease management system we need to keep in mind the simplicity of a desirable health care relation: it's a bi-directional relation of care, always available, always findable—as a matter of fact you don't have to look for it, it looks for you. One has a sense of being inside caring, of being nested in care— there's someone to turn to, to talk to, they suggest a few things to do, you do them, you turn to them again.

The protection of this simple relation, of its friendly permeating steadfast thoughtful presence, is the primary function of any system/culture built around it. Thus the system/culture would be so designed that this relation is either freely offered or offered at a low cost (supported by communal and social structures in a variety of ways); that the formation of any bureaucracy around it would be a sign of malfunctioning or predators, and steps would be taken to eliminate that; that creativity and variety would go into the design of the supporting nest into which the relation is put, and into the relation itself. So einfach.

5. Do we attempt to work with market institutions to change health care? Organized business is interested in discussing financing and administration, not health or health care. Thus, to sit down at the table with these major players in health care industries means to sit down

with people who frame every discussion of health/health care as a discussion of money and administration. If any other consideration is brought up, they will look at you with a patronizing eye—after all, they know their business—and turn it back into a discussion of financing. So we *can* sit down with them at the table, but we have to realize we're sitting down with opponents to any direction of creating a desirable health care system available to all.

6. We need to garner support from business people, on a person-by-person basis, for hands-off-health-care initiatives. To appeal to faith communities whose morals lead them to ethical political positions. Every businessman has his fatherhood looking over his shoulder; has his son-hood, brother-hood. Every businesswoman is also a mother, daughter, sister, friend. Do they want to overhear, in the waiting room, that cutting costs was a factor in why their grandchild died on the operating table? At some point in their lives, someone they care about will be in the system too. Their own pricey insurance policies cannot be transferred to everyone they care about.

7. We consider what is happening to health care in the US a local version of the same market theories that initiated Structural Adjustment Programs across the globe by WTO and World Bank. (Structural adjustments' primary focus is to shape institutions/countries so that they're attractive to long distance investment capital.)

Structural adjustment policies have been tried in South America, and met, in an increasing number of cases, with resistance. Let's link our resistance to structural adjustment policies at home to the resistance made by allies across the globe who are also fighting these policies.

Final Remarks

The components of what we're calling 'Whole System Design' are two calls: one is a call for a variety of designs of those elements that will be become the culture of health care; and the second is a call for the sentiment: "hands off health care, big business" to become infectious in the Americas. Both these calls are efforts to perturb the current system.

In 2006, people in the United States have a diagnosis of the problem of our health care system that is clear and intelligent. If you read blogs/letters/emails from the common person they articulate their discontent with the health care system in a sophisticated way. (See membership polls conducted in spring, 2006, by MoveOn.Org). People want a fundamental change in the health care system. This means, we want a change in the fundamentals.

We need to be prepared for the language/framing in response to this desire for change. When Medicare Plan D came out in May 2006, it was a 122-page document with lots of complicated sections, written for older Americans, telling them how to get pharmaceutical drugs. 122 pages? Huh? How was this allowed? Did the writers lack schooling, lack funding, lack time to do a better job? We don't think so. Plan D was a linguistic display of 'passive intervention'.

We need to watch out. The existing players (entrenched industries, along with their current protectorate: the government) will respond to our clear desire for fundamental change with an engineered Tower of Babel. The column of language is coming at us now: fundamental change in the health care system is re-framed as the question "who will pay for this expensive system?" as a debate between various complicated payment schemes, as a mandate for consumer choice. 'Universal insurance' will be used, to confuse us into thinking this means 'single payer'. The language will befuddle us, discourage us.

The temptation will be to leave the discourse around health care to the experts. They seem to know what they're talking about, right? None of these experts will challenge the structural power of the entrenched industries, the huge salaries of the health care corporations CEO's, the fact that pharmaceutical corporations top the chart for profit returns, etc.

Will we permit 'passive intervention', again? The statistic is cited, over and over again, that in the richest country in the world, nearly 48 million Americans do not get health care.

We say that in the richest country in the world, 300 million Americans do not get health care. Yes, of these 300 million, many people do get into the disease management bureaucracy, as they have insurance. But what is happening inside the medical system is no longer care; the 567,000 licensed doctors are not permitted to doctor; the 2.4 million nurses are being thwarted at nursing. The culture of health care in America is being morphed into something else.

When hospitals and clinics are businesses, and doctors/nurses become business people, who will we then turn to for health care?

November, 2006" [Dr Susan Parenti]

****

> 'A library is a hospital for the mind'.
> Anonymous

16 FURTHER READING

History of Mental Illness

J Andrews, J Briggs et al — The History of Bethlem
A history of the earliest of the Asylums.

Michel Foucault — Madness and Civilization
Interesting read on parallels between mental illness and historical beliefs.

Roy Porter — A Brief History of Madness
An easy-to-read history of mental illness and its treatment.

A Rogers — Behavioural Sciences & the Law
A paper around treatment with ECT

Sainsbury Centre for Mental Health — Beyond the Water Towers
Papers on aspects of the treatment of mental illness, from asylums to the present day. Very readable.

History of Mental Illness - Websites

http://bethlemgallery.com/event/unescorted-6/
Link toe Bethlem gallery, periodically open to the public

http://www.channel4.com/programmes/bedlam/articles/all/from-bedlam-to-slam-a-timeline
Timeline from Channel 4 of the history of mental illness

http://medhist.ac.uk/index.html
Wellcome Trust's website - history of mental illness

http://www.sciencemuseum.org.uk/broughttolife/themes/menalhealthandillness.aspx
The Science Museum, history of mental illness

Mental Health Charities

http://www.depressionalliance.org/
Mental health generally

http://www5.who.int/mental_health/main.cfm?p=0000000149
World Health Organization – mental health section

http://www.sane.org.uk/
SANE & saneline (helpline) mental health charity website

http://www.rethink.org/
Rethink (formerly National Schizophrenia Fellowship) mental health charity

http://www.retreat-hospital.org/
The Retreat hospital. Care for anyone with mental health problems (York Retreat)

www.turning-point.co.uk
Turning Point, for mental health rehabilitation & counselling

www.mind.org.uk
MIND, the mental health charity

GLOSSARY

A
activity therapy	treatment based on work, learning or play
acupuncture	therapy with needles for balancing energy
affective disorders	problems with mood
alleviate	relieve the symptoms of
alternative medicine	alternatives to drug therapies
Alzheimer's	Degenerative mental disease
Analysand	a person who attends for psycho analysis
Analytical Psychology	psychological therapy by Carl Jung
anatomy	the study of the human body
ancestor worship	culture of venerating dead ancestors
Apothecary	[historic] Pharmacist [Druggist, Chemist]
Approved SWorker	[ASW] detains under Mental Health Act
archetype	character trait (Jungian theory)
Asylum	Literally 'place of refuge'.
Auto hypnosis	Self hypnosis

B
BAC	British Association for Counselling
behavioural therapy	therapy modifying behaviour (actions)
Bethlem Asylum	2nd oldest Hospital in England
bile (black bile)	'humour'; responsible for depression
blood letting	historic treatment for mental illness
brain fever	historic term describing psychosis
Breuer Joseph	Victorian practitioner of hypnosis
Brief therapy	problem solving therapy

C
Causal factor	a trigger to an event
Community Care Act	legislation for closure of Asylums
care plan	written document, outlining care
Catharsis /cathexis	mental release
Cerebral palsy	Brain disease
Charcot Jean Martin	Victorian hypnotist before Freud
Chemist	scientist who prepares medications
Chymist	historic term - Pharmacist
Clinical Psychologist	Psychologist in medical setting
clinical responsibility	responsibility for patient care
CMHT	Community Mental Health Team
cognitive-behavioural	therapy of behaviour change
cohort	group with common characteristics
collective unconscious	[Jung]. Seat of ancestral myths

complementary therapies	therapies not based on medicine
conditioned response	behaviour depends upon stimulus
conflict (mental)	two or more opposing events
conscious (mind)	part of the mind aware of actions
Contra indication	Medication which reacts with another
construct	a given or set of givens
counselling	one of the talking cures
Counsellor	talking cure
crippled	[historic term] physically disabled
curse	wishing death or evil upon another

D

DBT	Dialectical Behaviour Therapy
Déjà vu	prior memory of an event
demon	devil or evil spirit
depot	a long lasting injection
depressive	[derogatory] term for depressive illness
depressive illness	Imbalance in brain chemistry
dissertation	essay at degree level
drive	energy or pull
Druggist	[historic] - Pharmacist
drugs	Medication, pharmaceuticals
dual diagnosis	physical & mental illness

E

Electro Convulsive Therapy	(ECT) electric shock treatment for chronic depression or schizophrenia
electric eels	[historic] treatment for madness
electro-encephalograph	brain activity reading machine
epilepsy	Failure of brain circuit; causes fits
ethical	moral code in a particular situation
eugenics	quasi science from Morel degeneration theory
evidence-based medicine	proven through research
evil spirits	entities blamed for madness
existential	to do with existence, life
extrovert	outgoing, confident personality

F

forensic psychiatry	criminal illness e.g. psychopathic
formulate	making of medications/ pills
free association	Freudian - meaningful connections
Freud Sigmund	Founder of psycho analysis
frontal lobes	area of brain for personality and mood

G

General Practitioner	doctor in a general practice
genetic factor	attributed to inherited
Green Paper	proposals for changes to legislation,
Group Home	homes for ex- patients living together
group therapy	One therapist & several patients

H

halo effect	Perception based on hearsay
hero	archetype - birth, death & resurrection
Hippocrates	Greek Philosopher who studied mind
humours / vital fluid	Ancient belief in four life-giving fluids
Hypno-Psychotherapist	therapist of brief therapy + hypnosis
hypnosis	Way of bypassing conscious mind
hypnotic state	state of relaxation [see trance]

I

idiot [historic term]	[historic] anyone with mental illness
Independent subscriber	staff who can prescribe without GP
individuation	Jungian concept of becoming unique
insanity	Mal functioning mental processes
institutionalization	deterioration of independence
introspective	Person who looks inward; reflective
introvert	Quiet type B personality

J

Jung CG	founder of Analytical Psychology
Jungian Analyst	follower of the Jungian school

L

Laing R. D.	psychiatrist who believed mental illness was a social condition
lay person	someone not formally trained
Lazar House	[historic] refuge house for lepers
laudanum	soporific drug
leech	Blood sucking worm
leucotomy (lobotomy)	psychosurgery, cutting frontal lobes
learning disability	intellect damaged due to brain damage
'liquid cosh'	[slang] medications dampening mood
lobotomy	see leucotomy
locum	temporary doctor acting for GP
lunatic	[historic] mad [comes from 'lunar']

M

mad	[historic] mentally ill
Madhouse	[historic] Asylum
madness	[slang] mental illness
maniac	[slang] psychopathic

manic	extreme excitement
MBBS	doctorate conferred on GPs
melancholia	[historic] depressive illness
mental defective	[historic] - see 'social misfit'
mental handicap	[historic] brain damage
Mental Health Act 1983	law for treatment of mentally ill
Mental Health Bill 2004	proposed legislation for mentally ill
Mental Health Tribunal	empowered to detain/ release patients
Mental Health Team	workers from different professions
Mental Health Worker	Graduate working in mental health
mental illness	illness of the mind
Mental Nurse	Nurse administering psychiatric drugs
metaphor	symbol or myth
Milton Erickson	American psychiatrist - brief therapy
Mind	national mental health charity
Moral panic	moral virtue of the moment

N

Nature /nurture	environment or upbringing?
neurosis	high anxiety state
NICE	Natl. Inst. of Clinical Excellence
NLP	brief therapy method

O

on-the-job training	training by working in field
Organic [disease]	Physical, not mental, damage
Orwell, George	Victorian social author

P

pathology [ical]	the course of an illness
Pavlov, Ivan Petrovich	Neurologist - conditioned response
Pharmacist	scientist who prescribes drugs
Phineas Gage	Victorian railworker
phrenology	[historic] character read from head
placebo effect	effect of belief on recovery
Primary Care Team	G.P.s / therapists in G.P. Practice
prognosis	expected outcome [medical]
Project 2000	Nurse training programme
Project Atlas (WHO)	mapping mental health resources
psyche	human soul or mind; Greek goddess
psychiatric hospital	hospital for the care of the mentally ill
Psychiatrist	Doctor with qualification in Psychiatry
psychiatry	treatment & study of mental disorders
psycho analysis	Sigmund Freud; study of the mind
Psycho Analyst	therapist; practices psycho-analysis

psychology	study of human behaviour
psychosurgery	brain surgery
Psychotherapist	therapist using talking cure for insight
purge (verb)	[historic] enema; historic 'cure'
Purposeful activity	activities to promote health.

R

refer	to introduce a patient
Rehabilitation Officer	therapist in the community
Rehabilitation Units	therapeutic community / hospital
remedy	cure or therapy; holistic medicine
research	systematic study to add knowledge
Responsible Medical Officer	Doctor delegated to oversee patient detained under the Mental Health Act
restraint	[historic] strait jacket; confines patient
rite (or ritual)	ceremony to mark life changes
ritual (in illness)	repetition of an act of cure or magic
Royal College of Psychiatrists	UK professional body of Psychiatrists

S

sanity	distinguish between real & imagined
Scapegoat	sacrificed animal or person
'schizo'	[slang] patient with schizophrenia
schizophrenia	illness of delusions & hallucinations
School of Thought	a particular method of training
section /sectioning	[slang] detain under Mental Health Act
sedative	drug to calm nervous system
self hypnosis	deep relaxation
session	therapeutic hour; 45mins – 1 hr
Shadow	Jungian archetype; evil or dark side
shaking palsy	[historic] for epilepsy or Parkinson's
Ship of Fools	[historic] mentally ill sent to sea
Skinner, Burrus Frederic	Scientist - behavioural theory
sleep & light temple	Roman therapy for depression
social housing	Low cost social housing
social integration	becoming part of society
social misfit	[historic] prostitute, tramp, thief
Social Worker	therapist of social orientated problems
solution-focused therapy	brief duration therapy
Spanish Inquisition	[Medieval] delegated to try witches
speaking in tongues	babbling; supposed voice of God
stigma	negative view through little knowledge
stimulant	drug or remedy which revives
strait jacket	[historic] canvas jacket with straps

subconscious	Part of mind out of our awareness
Supervisor (therapy)	Therapist trainer
supervision	learning through experienced therapist
supplementary prescriber	Specialist staff who prescribe
symbol[ic]	see metaphor, myth
symptom	sign of an illness
Szasz Thomas Dr	Psychiatrist of myth of mental illness

T

talking cure	therapies use talking as a cure
Mental Health Act	Enforced care of seriously mentally ill
Therapeutic Community	Community of patients and therapists
'therapeutic hour'	30 minutes to 45 minutes
Thorndike, Edward	Behaviourist - reward & responses
trepanning	primitive psycho-surgery
Tribunal	Committee; professionals and lay
'tuberculosis look'	[historic] pale & dark eyed

U

UKCP	Conference for Psychotherapy
unconscious	part of mind hidden from awareness

V

vital fluids	see 'humours'
voodoo and witchcraft	cult practised in Haiti

W

warrant	legal document for arrest or entry
Watson, John	Psychologist - learned behaviour
White Paper	Legal proposals from Government
Wise Old Man (Woman)	archetype; wisdom
Witch	[historic] servant of the devil
witchcraft	magic, for good or evil purposes
witch hunt	[historic] – scapegoat
witch mark	[historic] nipple where imps suckled
World Health Organization (WHO)	consortium of countries who come together to improve healthcare

ABOUT THE AUTHOR

Marianne Richards holds a Masters Degree in Mental Health Practice, Diploma in Ericksonian (Solution-Focused) Therapy & Certificate in Behavioural Family Therapy, as well as a media qualification. She worked for two decades in private practice and the NHS as Counsellor and Mental Health Worker, gaining praise from patients and Doctors. In 2000 she was offered her first publishing contract and subsequently received professional acclaim for her layman guides to adult mental illness.

Her life includes personal experience of mental illness which gives her books an extra dimension. Bullied out of the NHS, Marianne was diagnosed with depression and subsequently endured a breakdown. She was then diagnosed with high functioning autism, stress having triggered the florid symptoms which enabled diagnosis. These experiences inform her writing.

INDEX

A

Anti Psychiatric Movement, 40
archetypes, 33
Assertive Outreach, 50
Asylum, ix, 7, 8, 16, 22, 25, 27, 35, 36, 37, 46, 48, 107, 109
Asylum Buildings, Disposal, 44

B

Bethlehem. *See* Bethlem Hospital
Bethlem Hospital, v, 8, 10, 16
bloodletting, 16
Brief Therapy, 38

C

Charcot, 26, 32, 109
collective unconscious, 33, 109
Community Mental Health Team, 50
Contributory Factors to Mental Illness, 87
Country of the Blind, 2

D

David Bennett Report, 78
Degeneration - Morel, 27
Diagnosis, 78, 84
Dialectical behaviour therapy, 39
DR SUSAN PARENTI, 99
DSMV (diagnostics and statistics manual, 89

E

Early Intervention For Psychosis Team, 50
Electro Convulsive Therapy (ECT), v, 8, 16, 36, 39, 40, 57, 59, 64, 65, 107, 109
Emergency Duty Team, 50
Employability, 88
Encounter groups, 38
Erickson, Milton, 38
Exclusion. *See* stigmatization

F

Freud Sigmund, 13, 26, 32, 35, 39, 109
Further reading, 107

G

Glossary, 109
Graduate Mental Health Workers, 50, 53

H

Hippocrates, 7, 13, 30, 40, 41, 109
History of Mental Illness, 107
How a Bill Becomes Law, 67
humours, 14, 16, 109
Hutu and Tutsi tribes, 85

I

Inquisition, 19, 109

J

Jung Carl, 26, 32, 33, 34, 35, 39, 40, 109

L

Laing, R D, 40
Language of Stigma, 94
Lazar Houses, 7, 22
Leeches, 16
Living in Communities, 71
Lobotomy, 36, 41
Low Self Esteem, 86

M

Mad, Bad or Criminally Insane, 3
mandela, 16
marginalization, 1
melancholy, 13, 30
Mental Capacity Act 2005, 68
Mental Health Act 1983, i, 54, 61, 64, 109
Mental Health Act 2007, 68
Mental Health Bill 2004, 60
Mental Health Education, 89
Misunderstanding, 88
moral justice, 11
Myth of the House of Agamemnon, 13

N

NEW MODEL HEALTH CARE SYSTEM FOR THE US, 99
NHS & Community Act, 44

P

Pavlov Ivan, 35
Phineas Gage, 30
Plato, 16
psychiatric hospital, 46, 55, 109
Psychiatry, 26, 27, 109
purging, 16, 25

R

Rachel's Challenge, 97
Rake's Progress, 24
Rehabilitation Units, 48

S

Samaritans, 50
Sanity, 1, 5
Scapegoats, 91
Ship of fools, 22
Social Exclusion, i, 90, 93
stigmatization, 63, 78, 79
Sykes, Dr Kathy, 38
Symbolic Language, 93

T

talking therapy, 39
temporary work, 86
token economy, 37
Trepanning, 7, 11

V

Victoria Climbie Report, 74
Virtual Brains, 41

W

witchcraft, 19, 74, 76, 109
World Health Organization (WHO), 69

Y

York Retreat, 26

Z

zero hours contracts, 86

Printed in Great Britain
by Amazon